FROM FATIGUED TO FANTASTIC!

Jacob Teitelbaum, MD

AVERY PUBLISHING GROUP
Garden City Park • New York

The author and publisher do not advocate the use of any particular form of health care, but believe that the information presented in this book should be available to the public. This book is not intended to replace the advice and treatment of a physician. Any use of the information set forth herein is entirely at the reader's discretion.

Because there is always some risk involved, the author and publisher are not responsible for any adverse effects or consequences resulting from the use of any of the preparations or procedures described in this book. Please do not use this book if you are unwilling to assume the risk. Each person and situation is unique, and a physician or other qualified health care professional should be consulted if there is any question regarding the presence or treatment of any abnormal health condition. It is a sign of wisdom, not cowardice, to seek a second or third opinion.

Cover design: William Gonzalez
In-house editor: Elaine Will Sparber
Typesetter: Bonnie Freid

Avery Publishing Group, Inc.
120 Old Broadway
Garden City Park, NY 11040
1-800-548-5757

ISBN: 0-89529-896-1

Printed in the United States of America

10 9 8 7 6 5 4 3 2

Contents

*To my daughter, Amy; son, David;
mother, Sabina; and father, David,
whose unconditional love made this book possible.
And to my patients, who have taught me
more than I can ever hope to teach them.*

Acknowledgments

So many special people helped make this book possible that I cannot possibly list them all. In truth, I have created nothing new. I have simply synthesized the wonderful work done by an army of hard-working and courageous physicians and healers.

I would like to extend my sincerest thanks to:

First and foremost, my staff. Their hard work, compassion, and dedication (and, I must admit, patience with me) are what made my work possible.

My research partner and lab manager, Birdie (Barbara Bird). Her sense of humor and encouragement kept me going when I got tired. Her dedication to quality showed in every facet of her work.

Pat Miller, who was especially gracious. She made sure that everything went as smoothly as possible.

The Anne Arundel Medical Center librarian, Joyce Richmond. Over the last fifteen years, I have often wondered when she would politely tell me to stop asking for so many studies. So far, she has not. In fact, she always smiles when I ask her for more.

My transcriptionist, Laurie Spangler, C.M.T. She patiently put up with my mumbling and repeated rewrites.

My physician associates. Dr. Robert Greenfield taught me healthy skepticism, and Dr. Alan Weiss always reminded me to reclaim my sense of humor.

My publisher, Rudy Shur, and my editors, Elaine Will Sparber and Judith O'Callaghan. They guided me through unknown terrain.

My many teachers, the real heroes and heroines in their fields, whose names could fill this book. They include William Crook, Max Boverman, Brugh Joy, Janet Travell, William Jeffries, David Simons, Jay Goldstein, Paul Levine, Jorge Fletchas, I. Jon Williams, Leo Galland, the MAIP group, Leonard Jason, George Mitchell, Lloyd Lewis, Fletch Bartholomew, Michael Rosenbaum, Murray Susser, Paul Cheney, Alexander Chester, James Brodsky, Melvin Werbach, Sherry Rogers, Byron Hyde, Robert Ivker, Jeff Bland, Alan Gaby, and Jonathan Wright.

The many chronic fatigue syndrome and fibromyalgia support groups. These are easily the best patient support groups I have ever seen.

And finally, God and the universe, for the guidance and infinite blessings I have been given and for my role as an instrument for healing.

Preface

A curious thing happened during the rigorous process I went through to become a physician. By the time I completed my formal training, I presumed that if an important treatment existed for an illness, I had been taught about it. I understood that physicians need to keep reading to stay abreast of new information. But I *knew* that if someone claimed he or she could effectively treat a nontreatable disease, that person was a quack. If such a treatment existed, I would surely have been taught about it.

I was wrong.

Dr. Werner Barth, my rheumatology instructor, taught me many things. The most important thing he taught me, though, was to spend an hour a day reading the scientific literature. This has gotten me into all kinds of trouble.

When I first started my practice, patients would ask me if I knew about certain herbal or nutritional treatments for illnesses. One patient asked me if I had ever heard about using vitamin B_6 to treat carpal tunnel syndrome. "That's nonsense," I answered. "If B_6 cures carpal tunnel syndrome, don't you think I would have been taught to use that instead of to operate on people's wrists?" I said that I would look into it, however.

Joyce Richmond, the Anne Arundel Medical Center librarian, has always been happy to obtain studies for me (and she has gotten thousands over the years). When she did a literature search for vitamin B_6 and carpal tunnel syndrome, she found a number of studies showing that 250 milligrams of B_6 per day for three months combined with wrist splints often cures carpal tunnel syndrome. I thought that was curious. Over the months, this scene was played out again and again. I decided to keep notes on these rare "pearls" in a thirty-page spiral notebook. My notes are now over a thousand pages long.

After a while, I began to comprehend that, indeed, my professors had not taught me everything in medical school. As I continued my research, I realized that although our modern allopathic medical system might be the best in the world, it has its weaknesses. These days, it is rare (albeit wonderful) for a major medical development to come out of a doctor's office instead of a research center. This stems from a critical drawback to our economic system (and all systems have their drawbacks). In our current system, a treatment must be very profitable to be promoted. Experts estimate that it costs about $400,000,000 to develop a single new treatment and to get it through the Food and Drug Administration (FDA) approval process. Unless a medication or supplement is put through the FDA approval process, its manufacturer is banned from making any medical claims for the product. However, if a product is inexpensive and *nonpatentable*, its manufacturer will most likely not want to pay $400,000,000 to put it through the FDA process.

Vitamin B_6 used for carpal tunnel syndrome is an excellent example. Treating carpal tunnel syndrome with B_6 costs about $9 per patient. Vitamin B_6 manufacturers would therefore find it impossible to recoup the cost of getting FDA approval for this treatment. Because of this, most patients instead spend between $2,000 and $4,000 to have surgery. This situation is the same for hundreds of other nonpatentable, effective, inexpensive, and relatively safe treatments. The FDA has even been fighting to make it illegal for stores that sell supplements to hand out copies of well-done scientific studies on the supplements!

The treatment approach that you will learn about in *From Fatigued to Fantastic!* is well grounded in the scientific literature. Dr. Janet Travell, professor emeritus of internal medicine at George Washington University Medical School, is considered the world's leading expert on muscle disorders. She served as White House physician for presidents John F. Kennedy and Lyndon B. Johnson and authored the eight hundred–

page bible on treating muscle disorders entitled *Myofascial Pain and Dysfunction: The Trigger Point Manual*. Although the research connecting fibromyalgia and myofascial (muscle) pain syndromes had not yet been done when she wrote her book, she investigated the perpetuating factors—that is, the conditions that keep the muscles from appropriately relaxing. In one chapter alone, she referenced 317 scientific studies that showed how important it is to treat these perpetuating factors. There is no lack of scientific basis for treatment, just a lack of awareness of the treatment, due to its relative inexpensiveness and nonpatentability.

Unfortunately, your doctor is likely to be unfamiliar with the research on effective treatment of myofascial pain and fibromyalgia. Your doctor may be hostile to the information presented in this book, considering it to be quackery because it was not covered in medical school. Or, your doctor may choose to disregard the information. On the other hand, your doctor might be open-minded (though reasonably skeptical) and will choose to explore the subject in more depth. If this last possibility is the case, the information and references in this book will give your doctor the scientific basis necessary to manage and optimize your treatment. Show your doctor Appendix A: For Physicians, which I wrote specifically for medical professionals. Appendix B: Effective Treatment of Severe Chronic Fatigue: A Report of a Series of 64 Patients, in which I present the results that my research partner and I obtained in a recently published study, will also be helpful to your physician.

The book in general, however, is for you, the layperson suffering from chronic fatigue syndrome or fibromyalgia. After giving an overview of the possible causes and patterns of chronic fatigue states in Chapter 1, I hone in on the specifics. In Chapter 2, I discuss nutritional problems. In Chapter 3, I focus on hormonal problems. In Chapter 4, I cover immune-system problems and infections, and in Chapter 5, I discuss fibromyalgia. In Chapter 6, I address food allergies, sinus problems, sleep disorders, and several other possible troublemakers. In Chapter 7, I hope to convince you that you are not crazy, that your symptoms are most likely real. And in Chapter 8, I try to help you find a physician who will treat you as a whole person, addressing both the physical and the psycho-spiritual issues inherent in illness. Several appendices offer additional or supporting information.

I think you will find the material presented in this book to be as exciting as my colleagues and I find it. Knowing how problematic brain fog can be, I have tried to keep the text concise and straightforward. However, if you finish the book and find yourself wishing for more information, check Appendix C: Recommended Reading, as well as the Bibliography. Between this book, my reference sources, and the books and articles I recommend for further reading, you should find the bulk of your most pressing questions answered.

Introduction

I remember 1975. I was in my third year of medical school, doing my pediatrics rotation. I had always excelled, proven by my finishing college in three years. Now I was the second youngest in a class of over two hundred medical students, and I was continuing to excel. My approach to life was to move quickly—"full speed ahead." But then a nasty viral illness hit me and made it hard for me to even get out of bed for my pediatrics lecture. I cannot forget walking into an auditorium full of medical students, the professor saying, "Teitelbaum, why are you . . . ?" As he said "late," I just about collapsed on the steps.

Although I was barely able to function, I spent the next four weeks working in the electron microscopy and research labs. The work I performed there was considered low-key, good tasks for a medical student trying to recuperate. By the end of the month, however, I was finding it impossible to get out of bed even by noon. I wanted to push forward and try harder. Though it was not what I wanted to hear, a piece of advice that one wise professor gave me was that this was not a time to push forward but a time to take a leave of absence and regroup. I am still thankful for this man's guidance.

My illness seemed to close a door to one chapter of my life and open up other doors to whole new possibilities of self-exploration. Taking off in my '65 Dodge Dart, I had the novel experience of having no agenda, no plans. I was to meet many teachers on my journey. Most importantly, I was taking time to get to know myself.

With my family's and friends' help and support and my own inner work, I recovered my energy and strength and went on to finish medical school and residency. Though I did well, I continued to intermittently suffer the many diverse symptoms seen in fibromyalgia. My experiences with chronic fatigue syndrome (CFS) and fibromyalgia left me with an appreciation of the impact of this illness. The symptoms that persisted—such as fatigue, achiness, poor sleep, and bowel problems—acted as the arena in which I learned how to help other people overcome the disease.

If you have chronic fatigue syndrome, fibromyalgia, or another disabling chronic fatigue state, you have been through a difficult journey. I remember being told that I was depressed. I *was* depressed. I was unable to function. Most people with chronic exhaustion have to struggle just to get compassion and understanding.

Building on what I have learned since 1975, I, along with Barbara Bird, my lab manager and research partner, recently completed a study of sixty-four patients with disabling chronic fatigue. Mrs. Bird and I had treated hundreds of other patients before the study, and we have treated many hundreds more since. The majority of our patients have been cured—that is, their symptoms are no longer a problem—with our treatment, while most of the remainder have shown significant, albeit incomplete, improvement. Only 4 percent have had no significant change. We have found that, on average, patients begin to feel better in less than seven weeks.[1]

If you suffer from CFS or fibromyalgia, this book will provide you with the tools and information you need to move beyond fatigue and into wellness. If you are a physician, it will teach you how to help—often dramatically—your patients with chronic exhaustion, including those frustrating cases in which no treatment has thus far been successful.

If you have researched chronic fatigue and immune dysfunction syndrome (CFIDS), you will find information here that is familiar, but you will also discover much that is new. For instance, Mrs. Bird and I have found that the key to eliminating chronic fatigue is to treat all of the underlying problems simultaneously. Most sufferers of chronic exhaustion have a mix of five or six underlying problems because of a vicious cycle in which each problem causes several others. You may have found some relief in the past by treating one, or a few, of these problems. I think you will be happily surprised at what happens when you treat all your underlying problems simultaneously.

Certainly, we still have much more to learn in this area. However, we have now crossed a threshold and can effectively treat the illness. Many patients still obtain significant but incomplete relief. As new information surfaces, more and more people will hopefully join the ranks of those who find their chronic fatigue state resolved with the proper treatment!

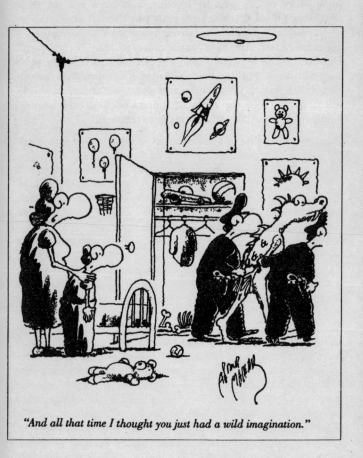

"And all that time I thought you just had a wild imagination."

1

What Is Chronic Fatigue Syndrome?

Chronic fatigue syndrome is a group of symptoms associated with severe, almost unrelenting fatigue. The predominant symptom is fatigue that causes a persistent and substantial reduction in activity level. Poor sleep, achiness, brain fog, increased thirst, bowel disorders, recurrent infections, and exhaustion after minimal exertion are some of the more common associated symptoms.

The Centers for Disease Control (CDC) has put together an updated list of criteria for chronic fatigue syndrome (see page 7). Although the CDC's criteria help researchers define groups for studies, its original criteria for chronic fatigue syndrome excluded all but about five thousand to twenty thousand people in the United States.[1-3] Unfortunately, three million to six million people in this country currently suffer from severe chronic fatigue states.[4] Research has shown that people with disabling fatigue who do not fit the CDC criteria have the same immunologic changes and responses to treatment as do those who do fit.[5] My experience, too, suggests that the underlying causes of patients' chronic fatigue and their responses to treatment are not affected by whether they strictly meet the CDC guidelines.[6] Therefore, I prefer to use the term *severe chronic fatigue states (SCFS)* for these conditions. The symptoms and tests described in this chapter will help you determine whether you have SCFS or another medical problem that requires a different treatment.

Patients who suffer from SCFS usually have a combination of several different problems. The exact combination varies from individual to individual. The major underlying factors number about twelve, with individual patients displaying an average of five to six factors each. It is important to look for and treat all of the factors simultaneously. Chronic fatigue states are unusual in that each separate problem can trigger other problems. Because of this, only one single underlying problem is rarely found by the time a patient seeks medical help.

To use an analogy, a person with a chronic fatigue state is like an automobile with a dead battery and a broken starter. If we only charge the battery, the car will not run. If we only repair the starter, the car will not run. However, if we both charge the battery and repair the starter, the car will be fine. In the same way, if we treat all of an SCFS patient's problems simultaneously, the person will feel well.

Common Patterns of Chronic Fatigue Syndrome

Several common subsets and patterns are seen in severe chronic fatigue states. They include what I call the drop dead flu, as well as fibromyalgia and the autoimmune triad.

THE DROP DEAD FLU

The most notorious pattern seen in severe chronic fatigue states is one in which a person who is feeling fine suddenly comes down with a brutal flulike illness that never goes away. The sudden onset of the illness after an infection is a mark of this classic pattern. In most CFS patients, an underlying viral infection is suspected.[7-10] This viral infection causes an inflammation in the brain that suppresses the hypothalamus gland.[11,12] Hypothalamic dysfunction is also common in chronic fatigue states.[13-17]

What happens when the hypothalamus gland is injured? The hypothalamus is the body's master gland. It controls most of the other glands, including the adrenal and thyroid glands. When it is suppressed, it in turn causes a subtle but disabling decrease in the functioning of many of the other glands. However, a person can experience fatigue and flulike symptoms just from suppression of the adrenal gland.

For most people, the suppression of the hypothalamus ends when the flu is over. Dr. William Jeffries, a Case-Western Reserve

Updated CDC Criteria for Chronic Fatigue Syndrome

A case of the Chronic Fatigue Syndrome is defined by the presence of the following:

1. Clinically evaluated, unexplained, persistent, or relapsing chronic fatigue that is of new or definite onset (has not been lifelong); is not the result of ongoing exertion; is not substantially alleviated by rest; and results in substantial reduction in previous levels of occupational, educational, social, or personal activities.

2. Concurrent occurrence of four or more of the following symptoms, all of which must have persisted or recurred during six or more consecutive months of illness and must not have predated the fatigue:

   A. Self-reported impairment in short-term memory or concentration severe enough to cause substantial reduction in previous levels of occupational, educational, social, or personal activities.

   B. Sore throat.

   C. Tender cervical or axillary lymph nodes.

   D. Muscle pain.

   E. Multijoint pain without joint swelling or redness.

   F. Headaches of a new type, pattern, or severity.

   G. Unrefreshing sleep.

   H. Postexertional malaise lasting more than 24 hours.

Adapted from the *Annals of Internal Medicine* 121 (14 December 1994).
Used with permission

University endocrinologist emeritus, has theorized that people who remain chronically ill after an infection have long-term, and at times permanent, hypothalamic-gland suppression. He has found that treating such patients with adrenal hormone (in doses that are normal for the body) can bring about marked improvement.[11] My research supports his findings.

What happens when the adrenal gland no longer functions properly? In severe cases, people have gone into shock and died from even minor stresses, such as dental work. In most cases, however, the suppression is less severe in both intensity and number of glands affected. Dr. Jeffries showed exactly what occurs in his excellent 1981 monograph, *Safe Uses of Cortisone.* He explained that the flu causes suppression of adrenocorticotropic hormone (ACTH), which is the hormone that causes the adrenal gland to make adrenal hormone. When the adrenal gland is suppressed—that is, when the adrenal gland does not make sufficient adrenal hormone—a variety of fatigue symptoms results. When Dr. Jeffries gave fatigue and flu patients low doses of adrenal hormone, the flulike symptoms often markedly improved.

Even though a gland is underactive, a blood test can show that it is technically normal, albeit in the low range.[13] This is why patients are often told that their thyroid or adrenal gland is healthy when indeed it is not. Because of this, doctors must know how to correctly interpret blood tests and how to identify subclinical hormonal deficiencies.

The drop dead flu also causes many patients to develop poor immunity, facilitating repeated bladder, respiratory, or sinus infections. I have found that patients who take repeated courses of antibiotics often end up with an overgrowth of yeast in the bowel. Bowel parasites, too, are common in CFS patients.[6] Suppressed thyroid or adrenal functioning and chronic infections can also trigger a problem called fibromyalgia.

FIBROMYALGIA

Fibromyalgia is basically a sleep disorder associated with shortened, achy muscles that have multiple tender knots. Trying to sleep on the tender knots is like trying to sleep on marbles. Because of this, people with fibromyalgia have trouble staying in the deep stages of sleep, which are the stages that recharge the batteries. Instead, these people stay in the light sleep stages and often wake up frequently during the night. They finally fall fast asleep just before the alarm clock is set to ring. In essence, fibromyalgia sufferers may not have slept *effectively* for several years. When normal sleep patterns are restored, they feel much better. Please note, however, that most sleeping pills—especially benzodiazepines, such as Valium, Halcion, and Dalmane—actually worsen deep sleep.

Fibromyalgia also causes fatigue by further suppressing the hypothalamus gland.[15] This results in immune suppression with secondary bowel infections. The bowel infections seen in chronic fatigue can cause decreased absorption of nutrients and may prompt increased nutritional needs, which in turn can lead to vitamin and mineral deficiencies. The hormonal and nutritional deficiencies cause the fibromyalgia to persist, and the fatigue cycle thus continues. (For a simplified illustration of this cycle, see Figure 1.1. For a more detailed illustration, see Figure A.1 on page 93.)

Many people enter the fatigue cycle directly through fibromyalgia. Fibromyalgia can be triggered by a trauma, such as an accident; a parasitic or other infection; or chronic emotional or physical stress. It can also be triggered by a number of other problems, such as an anatomic dysfunction (for example, legs of different lengths) or temporomandibular joint (TMJ) syndrome, which is characterized by tenderness and clicking in the jaw.

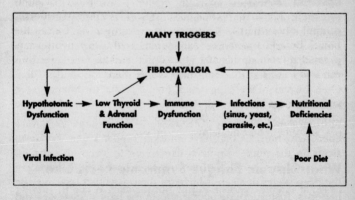

Figure 1.1. The fatigue cycle.

THE AUTOIMMUNE TRIAD

Another common pattern seen in severe chronic fatigue states is the autoimmune triad. In autoimmune disorders, the body mistakes parts of itself for outside invaders. The autoimmune triad seen in CFS patients involves the thyroid and adrenal glands as well as the cells in the body that assist in the absorption of vitamin B_{12}. When the body attacks these "invaders," the resulting low thyroid, adrenal, and B_{12} levels trigger fibromyalgia, which then suppresses the hypothalamus gland, which sets the fatigue cycle in motion.

IS THE PATTERN IMPORTANT?

Many patients fit into one of the three patterns just described, but many patients do not. Many other patterns also exist. When I ask patients when their problems began, I sometimes get an answer to the exact date—year, month, and day. These patients usually fall into the first category because they had an infection that suppressed the hypothalamus gland. Other people answer, "Oh, the problem began about three to four years ago." These people most often fall into the second category, with fibromyalgia as the predominant factor, perhaps accompanied by an underlying yeast or parasitic infection in the bowel. However, they also commonly fall into the third category—the autoimmune triad.

Sometimes, the exact pattern cannot be determined, and to be honest, it often does not really matter. I now treat the entire process at once so that my patients can recover more quickly. This method has its trade-offs, though. By treating several processes simultaneously, I sometimes cannot tell exactly which treatment is producing the main benefit. However, I feel that treating two to three processes at the same time works more efficiently. Then, when the patient is feeling better, I taper off the treatments to see which ones are still needed. Regarding your treatment, the choice of whether to treat two to three problems simultaneously or only one at a time is best made by you and your physician.

What Chronic Fatigue Syndrome Feels Like

Chronic fatigue syndrome and fibromyalgia occur in varying degrees of severity. Many people have mild to moderate fatigue with achiness and poor sleep. Often, these people attribute the symptoms simply to aging or stress. Others have fatigue so disabling that they cannot even get out of bed, let alone participate in regular day-to-day activities.

The most common complaints that chronic fatigue and fibromyalgia patients have are:

- *Overwhelming fatigue.* Most people with CFS are fatigued most or all of the time. Occasionally, they have periods—that is, short spans of time lasting for several hours or days—during which they feel better. However, what they usually try to do during those good periods is make up for lost time. What they end up doing is crashing and burning.

  Most CFS patients wake up tired. This is especially true of fibromyalgia patients. In addition, exercise often makes the fatigue worse. When CFS patients try to exercise, they feel more fatigued later that day and usually feel as if they were hit by a truck the next day. This causes further deconditioning and discouragement.

- *Frequent infections.* Many CFS patients have recurrent sinus or respiratory infections, sore throats, swollen glands, bladder infections, or vaginal, bowel, or skin yeast infections. Some have a recurrent red, bumpy rash that is resistant to treatment. They often find that this rash goes away for the first time in years when they have their bowel fungal overgrowth treated. Abdominal gas, cramps, and bloating are also very common, as is alternating diarrhea and constipation. These digestive complaints are attributed to spastic colon and are often triggered by bowel yeast or parasitic infections. Poor food absorption and food sensitivities may also play significant roles in the onset of bowel symptoms.

- *Brain fog.* Brain fog is almost routine. Chronic fatigue patients often suffer from poor memory and occasionally from confusion. Their minds may seem foggy. Brain fog is one of the most frustrating symptoms of CFS for some patients and is often the scariest. It is also a complaint that is routinely resolved with treatment.

- *Achiness.* Chronic diffuse achiness in both muscles and joints is also very common in chronic fatigue patients. For most, this achiness is part of their fibromyalgia. (For a discussion of the achiness associated with fibromyalgia, see Chapter 5.)

- *Increased thirst.* When I meet a new patient who has a water bottle in hand, I usually know what the main complaint will be. As part of their hormonal problems, people with chronic fatigue have increased urine output and, therefore, increased thirst. A classic description of these patients is that they "drink like a fish and pee like a racehorse." Drinking a lot of water is very important. In fact, many CFS patients find that they need to drink two to three times as much liquids as the average person. I recommend filtered water (see page 49.)

- *Allergies.* Fatigue patients often have a history of being sensitive to many foods and medications. They often get away with small doses of medications and respond adversely to normal or large doses. Fortunately, severe environmental sensitivity is much less common. I find that food and other sensitivities usually improve when the adrenal insufficiency and yeast or parasitic overgrowth are treated.

- *Anxiety and depression.* People with CFS not uncommonly have marked anxiety with palpitations, sweating, and other signs of panic. The CFS, combined with nutritional deficiencies, aggravates the tendency to anxiety and depression. These symptoms, too, often improve with treatment.

You may have recognized yourself as you read through this list. If you did, please be assured that you are part of a large group of people. You are not alone. Several excellent national support groups exist, including the Fibromyalgia Network and the Chronic Fatigue and Immune Dysfunction Syndrome Association of America. These are effective support groups, actively searching for answers to the CFS puzzle. Their addresses, as well as those of some other excellent local support groups and additional organizations, are in Appendix G: Patient Support Groups.

Many pieces of the CFS puzzle are still missing. The outlook is bright, however, with new research continually providing important clues to how to improve treatment. For the vast majority of people with CFS symptoms, effective treatment is now available.

Important Points

- Chronic fatigue patients usually have a variety of symptoms in addition to fatigue. Common ones are achiness, poor sleep, poor memory, brain fog, increased thirst, and frequent infections.

- Chronic fatigue usually has a *mixture* of underlying causes. This is because each problem can trigger other problems. For example, hormonal problems can trigger disordered immunity, which can trigger bowel yeast, parasitic, and other infections, which can trigger fibromyalgia, which can further worsen hormonal problems.

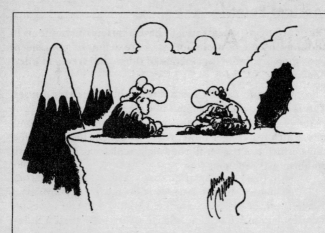

"It's the mystical balance of the universe. For every hotel towel you steal, a sock will disappear from your dryer."

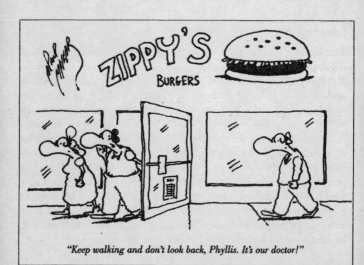

"Keep walking and don't look back, Phyllis. It's our doctor!"

2

Going After
the Easy Things First

Often, people come in complaining of long-standing fatigue that is not quite as disabling as what accompanies chronic fatigue syndrome or fibromyalgia. I never cease to be amazed at how often these people dramatically improve by simply cleaning up their diets a little—cutting down on their sugar, caffeine, and alcohol intakes; substituting whole grains for white flour; and adding a good multivitamin supplement to their daily regimens. So, let us start with the easy things first.

Sugar and White Flour

The average American's diet includes over 140 pounds of added sugar per year.[1] This added sugar accounts for 18 percent of the average American's caloric intake. Since a healthy diet without added sugar has only a 5- to 15-percent margin of safety for supplying optimum amounts of the vitamins and minerals, the added sugar alone makes the average American diet a disaster.

I often hear people express skepticism about the importance of nutritional supplements. A typical comment that I hear is, "Five hundred years ago, there were no vitamin tablets, and people seemed to do just fine." Well, five hundred years ago, sugar was expensive and not readily available. The king of England might have sprinkled a teaspoon of sugar on his food as a sign of power, but when he wanted sugar and had none left, he had to send someone to the West Indies to get it.

Another dietary disaster is white flour. Vitamins were supposedly discovered by a Dutch settler who went on sailing expeditions with Dutch explorers. Soon after the settler helped a group of colonists establish their new home, he found that the colonists were becoming ill. He also noticed that the colony's chickens were looking unusually healthy. Being a curious fellow, this man began feeding the chicken food to the people. Over a period of several weeks, the people became stronger and healthier. Since the settler was also a good businessman, he (incorrectly) named the chicken feed *vital amines*, meaning *vital proteins*, and began selling it. The name was later shortened to *vitamins*.

Today, scientists understand what happened to those colonists. Polishing off the brown outer coat, or bran, from rice had become fashionable. The rice bran was then used as chicken feed. The bran, however, is what contains most of the vitamins and minerals that are present in rice. The colonists therefore quickly became nutritionally deficient, while the chickens flourished.

In the United States, approximately 18 percent of the average person's calories come from white flour. However, white flour, just like white rice, has had the bran removed and therefore is also significantly depleted of vitamins and minerals.[1,2] Although some foods made of white flour are now fortified with vitamins and minerals to make up for this, *most* of the nutrients that were removed continue to be missing.

As you can see, from just the use of white flour and added sugar, Americans reduce their vitamin and mineral intake by up to 35 percent. Add to this the nutrients that are lost in the canning of vegetables, which can cause vitamin losses of up to 80 percent, and in the processing of other foods.[3] As Dr. S. B. Eaton noted in his study in the prestigious *New England Journal of Medicine*, "Physicians and nutritionists are increasingly convinced that the dietary habits adopted by western society over the past one hundred years make an important etiologic [causative] contribution to coronary heart diseases [angina], hypertension, diabetes, and some types of cancer."[4] This is the same conclusion that was reached by the authors of *Western Diseases: Their Emergence and Prevention.*[5]

It soon becomes obvious that the argument about people not needing vitamin tablets five hundred years ago does not apply to the average modern American. One study that was reported in the *American Journal of Clinical Nutrition* showed that less than 5 percent of the study participants consumed the recommended daily amounts (RDAs) of all the vitamins and minerals.[6] What is frightening is that this study was conducted in Beltsville, Maryland, on United States Department of Agriculture (USDA) research center employees.

Every vitamin and mineral is *very* important in some way to health. In addition, sugar nurtures the growth of yeast in the bowel and stimulates yeast overgrowth. Yeast grows by fermenting sugar, and it says thank-you by making billions of baby yeasties. Physicians working in this field have found that although most sugar is usually absorbed before it gets to the bowels, excess sugar can markedly aggravate yeast overgrowth.[7] (For a complete discussion of yeast overgrowth, see page 42.) Sugar can also aggravate hypoglycemia, which is commonly found in people with an underactive adrenal gland. (For a discussion of hypoglycemia, see page 29.)

Caffeine and Alcohol

I am constantly astonished over how many people who complain about being tired drink more than ten cups of coffee a day. Caffeine is a loan shark for energy. Many chronic fatigue patients fall into the trap of drinking ever-increasing amounts of coffee to boost their energy so that they can function. What these people do not realize is that as the day goes on, caffeine takes away more energy than it gives. Coffee drinkers are caught in a vicious cycle. I advise all my coffee drinkers to stop ingesting caffeine completely for two to three months. After this initial period, I tell them that they can add back *up to* ten ounces of coffee a day if they are feeling better.

If you drink more than three cups of coffee a day, you should remove it from your diet gradually. To begin, cut your coffee consumption in half every week until you are down to about one cup a day. For example, if you generally drink four cups of coffee a day, cut your intake to two cups a day the first week, then to one cup a day the second week. The final week, switch to tea with some caffeine. I usually tell my patients that I do not want to see them until ten days after their last cup of coffee. Caffeine is a drug and removing it from the diet brings withdrawal symptoms—grouchiness, headache, and fatigue. Once the withdrawal symptoms are gone, however, my patients usually feel much better and are very happy that they went through the process. By tapering the coffee as just described, it takes a little longer to feel well, but the withdrawal symptoms are not as severe.

Limit alcohol to one to two drinks a day. One drink equals six ounces of wine, twelve ounces of beer, or one and a half ounces of whiskey. If you drink more than these amounts, you should stop drinking alcohol completely for three months. If you decide to return alcohol to your diet at the end of that time, make two drinks a day your limit. Many people with fatigue find that even the smallest amount of alcohol is too much.

Vitamin and Mineral Supplements

The body is dependent on receiving vitamins and minerals from the diet because it cannot make them itself. Especially important are the B vitamins, iron, and magnesium. If you are low in vitamins and minerals—whether because you eat junk food and are not taking in the required nutrients or because you are consuming the proper foods but your body is unable to correctly metabolize them—your fibromyalgia simply will not subside. A good multivitamin supplement is therefore critical to your improvement.

Taking a multivitamin that supplies at least 25 milligrams each of vitamin B_1 (thiamine), vitamin B_2 (riboflavin), vitamin B_3 (niacin), and vitamin B_6 (pyridoxine), as well as good amounts of folic acid, vitamin B_{12}, and biotin and an adequate representation of minerals can have a dramatic effect on your well-being. I recommend that almost all my chronic fatigue patients take an excellent multivitamin called TwinLab Daily One Caps with iron. TwinLab Daily One Caps can be purchased in most health food stores or by mail order (see Appendix I: Mail Order Sources). I recommend this brand because all vitamins are not created equal and many are made very poorly. If you have a high risk of heart disease, such as a strong family history or a high cholesterol count, take the version without iron, unless your blood test shows that you are low in that mineral.

Why are vitamins and minerals so important? Dr. Janet Travell, White House physician for presidents John F. Kennedy and Lyndon B. Johnson and professor emeritus of internal medicine at George Washington University, cowrote *Myofascial Pain and Dysfunction: The Trigger Point Manual*, which is acknowledged as the authoritative work on muscle problems. In one chapter alone, Dr. Travell and coauthor Dr. David Simons reference 317 studies showing that problems such as hormonal, vitamin, and mineral deficiencies can contribute to muscle disorders.[8]

Numerous other studies have shown that adequate vitamins and minerals, especially folic acid and zinc, are critical for proper immune function—that is, for defense against infections. Vitamin A, beta-carotene, vitamin B_6, vitamin C, vitamin E, iron, and many other nutrients have also been found to be very important in keeping the body's defenses strong.[9-14]

Iron is important because an iron level that is too high or too low can cause fatigue,[15] poor immune function,[11,12,16] cold intolerance, decreased thyroid function, and poor memory.[17,18] I routinely recommend that all my chronic fatigue patients have their iron, total iron binding capacity (TIBC), and ferritin blood levels checked. These three tests all measure iron status. Some insurance companies balk at paying for all three tests, but the data and my clinical experience strongly support having them done. Even if a person's iron levels are just on the low side of normal, that person will often feel fatigued, despite not being anemic. Technically, the iron level is normal if the ferritin (iron storage) level is over 18. However, even minimal inflammation, such as a bladder infection, will falsely elevate the ferritin measurement and make it appear to be normal. This is why all three tests for iron deficiency are necessary.

One study reported in the British medical journal *Lancet* showed that infertile females whose ferritin levels were between 20 and 40—that is, technically normal—were often able to become pregnant when they took supplemental iron.[19] This suggests that levels considered normal to prevent anemia are often inadequate for other body functions. Because of this, anybody whose ferritin level is below 40, or whose percent saturation is less than 22 percent, should be considered a prime subject for a trial treatment of iron therapy.

A surprisingly high number of people also display early hemo-chromatosis on their iron studies. Hemochromatosis is a disease of excess iron. Early in the disease, fatigue is often the only symptom. If caught early, hemochromatosis is remarkably easy to treat. If caught late, however, it is disabling and fatal. This disease is an additional reason to check the iron level carefully.

Vitamin B_{12} is another key nutrient in CFS. Technically, the B_{12} level is normal if it is over 208 picograms per deciliter. However, studies have shown that people can suffer severe and sometimes long-term nerve and brain damage from B_{12} deficiency even if their levels are as high as 300 picograms per deciliter.[20] The question that arises then concerns why the normal levels are set so low. In part, they were initially set according to what prevents anemia. But the brain's and nervous system's needs for vitamin B_{12} are often much higher than those of the bone marrow. Also, as much as I hate to admit it, the medical establishment has greatly enjoyed poking fun at the old-time doctors who gave vitamin B_{12} shots for fatigue. The use of B_{12} shots despite "normal" levels is almost a symbol for unscientific, archaic medicine. As noted in an editorial in the *New England Journal of Medicine*, however, current findings suggest that those old-time doctors may have been right.[21] I suspect, though, that the modern medical establishment will be a little slow to eat crow.

Further proof comes from Japan, where, I have been told (although I have been unable to confirm it), a B_{12} level under 400 picograms per deciliter is often considered abnormal and treated. In other proof, a recent study using the respected Framingham Data Base showed that metabolic signs of B_{12} deficiency occur even with levels over 500 picograms per deciliter.[22] Furthermore, Alzheimer's victims have an average B_{12} level of only 472 picograms per deciliter, compared to people who have confusion from a non-Alzheimer's condition (such as a stroke), whose average B_{12} levels run 887 picograms per deciliter.[23] These and other studies suggest that many people need B_{12} levels that are significantly higher than what is currently considered normal.

In my experience, when their other problems are also treated, many people respond dramatically to B_{12} injections. If a patient's level is under 540 picograms per deciliter, I treat that person with a 1-milligram shot once a week. These shots are very safe and fairly inexpensive. Usually, if a patient is going to benefit from the shots, I see improvement by the seventh or eighth shot. I usually stop after eight to ten shots. If a patient's symptoms return after a few weeks, I resume giving the shots, usually every one to five weeks for an extended period of time. Most people, however, maintain their B_{12} level just by taking a multivitamin supplement.

Why is a low B_{12} level such a common problem in CFS patients? Several possibilities exist. Among them are the following:

- Vitamin B_{12} is important in the repair of nerve injuries. Evidence suggests that a process called myalgic encephalomyelitis occurs in the brain during the development of CFS. In repairing this injury, the body may overutilize vitamin B_{12} and, therefore, may overly deplete its stores.

- If an autoimmune process impairs the thyroid or adrenal gland, it often also decreases the body's ability to absorb vitamin B_{12}. (For a discussion of autoimmunity, see page 10.)

- Bowel overgrowth of yeast or parasites or problems with absorption may prevent the proper absorption of vitamin B_{12}.

Whatever the cause, I have found that treating patients with B_{12}, even if their levels are technically normal, often results in marked improvement.

In addition to a multivitamin supplement and B_{12} shots, I also urge my CFS patients to take a magnesium supplement. Magnesium is involved in over eighty-two different body functions but is routinely low in the American diet as a result of food processing. The average American diet supplies less than 300 milligrams of magnesium per day, while the average Asian diet supplies over 600 milligrams per day.[24,25] I generally recommend taking two 60-milligram tablets of magnesium chloride, magnesium lactate, or, preferably, magnesium malate two to three times a day. If diarrhea and cramps are not a problem, you can take up to twelve 60-milligram tablets a day. Six tablets per day will bring your dietary magnesium level just up to normal. If your magnesium is low, your muscles will stay in spasm and your fibromyalgia will not resolve. This is one of the reasons that taking magnesium is so critical. In addition, magnesium is important for the muscles' and body's strength and energy.[24] Take the magnesium for eight to ten months, since it may take this long to replace your deficits. Keep in mind that magnesium blood tests do not drop below normal until *severe* magnesium depletion occurs.[26]

If you do get diarrhea from the magnesium, cut the dosage back. Do not take magnesium if you have kidney failure—that is, if your creatinine level is over 1.6, which is very rare in chronic fatigue and immune dysfunction syndrome (CFIDS) patients. If your creatinine is 1.5 to 1.6, take just two 60-milligram tablets a day for two to three months. Before taking any magnesium, discuss your dosage and regimen with your physician.

Magnesium chloride and magnesium lactate are available over-the-counter at most pharmacies. I recommend Slow-Mag or Mag-Tab SR. If you ask for magnesium chloride at a health food store, you will probably pay less. Plain magnesium oxide is also available and is the most inexpensive form of magnesium. However, your body may not absorb it well. If you choose to take magnesium oxide, take 500 milligrams per day. The best form of magnesium is magnesium malate, which is available in health food stores as well as by mail order (see Appendix I).

The main side effect of multivitamins is an upset stomach, which occurs in only a small percentage of people. If this is a problem for you, try taking the vitamin with a meal or at bedtime. If the stomach discomfort persists, switch to another brand. I usually tell my patients to try a Centrum multivitamin supplement in the morning and a B-complex supplement in the afternoon or evening. If you still have problems, experiment until you find a brand of multivitamin that your stomach can tolerate. Please note that any supplement containing B vitamins will turn your urine bright yellow. This is normal.

Although I strongly recommend taking nutritional supplements to ensure obtaining the necessary nutrients, I also want to stress that eating a good healthy diet is important. Eat a lot of whole grains, fresh fruits, and fresh vegetables. Many raw vegetables have enzymes that help boost energy levels. You do not have to cut out all foods that might be bad or eat a diet that is impossible to follow. All that you need to do is eat a diet that is reasonably healthy and low in added sugar. The more unprocessed your diet is, the healthier you will be.

Important Points

- Remove sugar and other sweeteners from your diet.

- Use whole grain flour instead of white flour.

- Remove caffeine from your diet.

- Limit alcohol consumption to one or two drinks daily.

- Treat nutritional deficiencies with a daily multivitamin that has as least 25 milligrams each of vitamins B_1, B_2, B_3, and B_6.

- Treat a suboptimal iron level with an iron supplement. A high iron level also needs to be treated.

- Vitamin B_{12} shots can be very helpful in treating a vitamin B_{12} deficiency.

- Treat a magnesium deficiency with magnesium chloride, magnesium lactate, or, preferably, magnesium with malic acid.

- In addition to taking supplements, eat a healthy diet that includes lots of fresh fruits and vegetables and a minimum of processed foods.

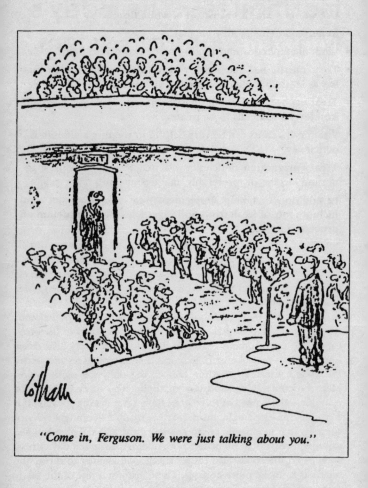

"Come in, Ferguson. We were just talking about you."

3

Hormones—The Body's Master Control System

The body's metabolism is controlled by a series of glands that create messengers called hormones. These hormones are controlled by feedback mechanisms that are interconnected and constantly interacting with one another in an elaborate dance. The dance is initiated by the hypothalamus, an ancient structure that is located deep inside the brain. The hypothalamus is the body's master gland and acts like the conductor in an orchestra. It sends hormones to its next-door neighbor, the pituitary gland, which in turn controls the thyroid gland, the adrenal glands, and the ovaries in females and testicles in males. The hypothalamus also monitors the levels of the hormones that all these glands make and tells the glands whether to make more or less.

Many factors determine how much hormone the hypothalamus directs each gland to make. A very mysterious gland in the brain called the pineal gland makes melatonin (and likely also other hormones, as yet unknown). I suspect that this gland also regulates the body's circadian rhythm—that is, the daily day-night cycles. Many functions in the body are rhythmic. The adrenal gland, for example, makes most of its cortisol hormones during the day. If it makes too much at night, the person has trouble sleeping. Evidence suggests that in chronic fatigue patients, the adrenal glands make too much cortisol at night and not enough during the day. Stress, such as an infection, also causes the hypothalamus to direct the adrenals to make more cortisol. These are just a few of the many factors that regulate hormone production.

Functions of the Different Glands

As just noted, the pineal, hypothalamus, and pituitary glands, located deep within the brain, work together to direct and balance the body's energy (the metabolic system) and defense (the immune system), as well as the part of the nervous system that controls blood flow to the skin, muscles, and organs (the autonomic-sympathetic-parasympathetic nervous systems). Current evidence suggests that a major portion of the symptoms of CFIDS and fibromyalgia are manifestations of a poorly functioning hypothalamus.

What roles do the different glands play? The thyroid gland is the body's gas pedal. It slows or speeds up the metabolism. If it is underactive, it causes fatigue, achiness, weight gain, poor mental functioning, and intolerance.

The adrenal glands are really several glands in one. They help direct the body's defense systems plus assist the body in dealing with stressful situations. If they are underactive, they cause fatigue, recurrent or persistent infections, hypoglycemia, allergies or environmental sensitivities, low blood pressure, dizziness, sugar craving, and poor ability to cope with stress.

The ovaries in females and the testicles in males support and cycle the reproductive system. The ovaries regulate menstruation in women, and both the ovaries and testicles contribute to libido (sexual desire). The male and female states of mind are powerfully influenced by the hormones produced by these glands. Although testosterone is known as the male hormone, it is also present in females. If either testosterone or the female hormone, estrogen, is low, the person may feel tired, depressed, weak, or moody. He or she may also feel a loss of libido and suffer from disordered sexual function and hot flashes.

Current research is increasingly demonstrating the dramatic role that suppression of the hormonal system plays in CFIDS and fibromyalgia. This chapter will present an overview of the latest research findings.

Adrenal Insufficiency

The adrenal glands, which sit on top of the kidneys, are actually two different glands in one. The center of the gland makes adrenaline (epinephrine) and is under the control of the autonomic nervous system. Although it is known that this part of the nervous system is also on the fritz in chronic fatigue patients—causing such symptoms as hot and cold sweats, cold sweaty hands, neurally mediated hypotension, and panic attacks—it is not understood if or how this ties into the adrenal's ability to make adrenaline. More likely, this is a central brain problem.

The outer part of the adrenal, the cortex, also makes many important hormones. These include:

- *Cortisol.* The adrenal glands increase their production of cortisol in response to stress. Cortisol raises the blood sugar and blood pressure levels and moderates immune function, in addition to playing numerous other roles. If the cortisol level is low, the person has fatigue, low blood pressure, hypoglycemia, poor immune function, an increased tendency to allergies and environmental sensitivity, and an inability to deal with stress.

- *Dehydroepiandrosterone-sulfate (DHEA-S).* Although its mechanism of action is not clear, DHEA is the most abundant hormone produced by the adrenal cortex. If low, the person feels poorly. Patients often feel dramatically better when their DHEA-S levels are brought to the midnormal range for a twenty-nine-year-old. DHEA levels normally decline with age, prompting many people to feel that this is one mechanism that the body uses to cause people to age and die to make room for newborns. DHEA levels appear to drop prematurely in chronic fatigue patients.

- *Aldosterone.* This hormone helps to keep salt and water balanced in the body.

- *Estrogen and testosterone.* These female and male hormones, respectively, are produced in small but significant amounts by the adrenals as well as by the ovaries and testicles.

About two-thirds of chronic fatigue patients appear to have an underactive adrenal gland. One reason may be that the hypothalamic master gland does not make enough corticotropin releasing hormone (CRH), which is the brain's way of telling the adrenal that more cortisol is needed. I suspect that many people also have adrenal burnout. Dr. Hans Selye, one of the first doctors to research stress reactions, found that if an animal becomes overstressed, its adrenal glands bleed and develop signs of adrenal destruction before the animal finally dies from the stress.

If you think back to your biology classes in high school, you may remember something called the fight or flight reaction. This is a physical reaction that occurs during times of stress. During the Stone Age, when a caveman met an animal that wanted to eat him, the caveman's adrenal glands activated multiple systems in his body that prompted him to either fight or run. This reaction helped the caveman survive. In those days, however, people probably had a couple of weeks or months to recover before facing the next major stress.

In today's society, people often experience stress reactions every few minutes. For example, when driving to work, a woman is delayed because of heavy traffic. While sitting behind the wheel, she frets about the consequences of her walking into the office late. Every time she hits a red light or pulls up behind a car that has slowed down, her adrenal gland's fight or flight reaction goes off again. When she finally arrives at work, she finds her boss waiting for her, which triggers the reaction once more. During the day, the woman may also have to deal with stresses such as angry customers or difficult coworkers. Her husband or children may phone, forcing her to deal with family stresses. If the woman is ill—suffering from CFS, for example— she has another major stress. The different problems associated with CFS, such as sinus infections and fibromyalgia, put more stress on her adrenal glands.

I suspect that many people suffer a burnout of their adrenal glands similar to the adrenal-gland destruction that Hans Selye saw in his experimental animals. With the kinds of stresses common in modern society, a person's adrenal test may show hormonal levels that are actually higher than usual, since the adrenal gland tends to overcompensate to deal with stress. The adrenal reserve—that is, the adrenal's ability to increase hormone production in response to stress—may be diminished, however. In endocrinologist Dr. William Jeffries' experience, and in mine as well, people with either low hormone production or a low reserve often respond dramatically to treatment with a low dose of adrenal hormone.[1,2]

Dr. Jeffries' opinion is that everyone who has unexplained disabling chronic fatigue should be given a low-dose trial of adrenal hormone.[3] Although Dr. Jeffries may well be on the mark, I tend to use this treatment first only on patients who fail the cortrosyn stimulation test, which tests adrenal function. However, the test can be interpreted in many different ways, and I tend to be a little more liberal than most when interpreting the results.

If your adrenal gland is underactive, what might you be experiencing? A low adrenal can cause, among other symptoms, the following:

- Fatigue.
- Recurrent infections.
- Difficulty shaking off infections.
- Poor response to stress.
- Achiness.
- Hypoglycemia.
- Low blood pressure and dizziness upon first standing.

Hypoglycemia deserves special mention. Many people sometimes become shaky and nervous, then dizzy, irritable, and fatigued. These people often feel better after they eat sweets, which improve their energy and mood for a short period of time. Because of this, these people often crave sugar, not realizing that it makes their blood sugar level initially shoot back up to normal, which is what makes them feel better, but then makes it continue shooting up beyond normal. Their bodies respond by driving the sugar level back down below normal again. The effect energywise is like a roller coaster.

Dr. Jeffries has noted—and again, my experience confirms his finding—that most people with hypoglycemia have an underactive adrenal gland. This makes sense because among the adrenal glands' responsibilities is maintenance of blood sugar at an adequate level. Sugar is the only fuel that the brain can use. When a person's blood sugar level drops, that person feels poorly.

Hypoglycemics can treat their low blood sugar symptoms by cutting sugar out of their diets; having frequent, small meals; and increasing their intake of complex carbohydrates such as whole grains and vegetables. Fruits—not fruit juices, which contain concentrated sugar—can be eaten in moderation, about one to two pieces a day, depending on the type of fruit. Taking 250 micrograms of glucose tolerance factor (GTF) chromium or chromium picolinate twice a day for six months often smoothes out hypoglycemic symptoms.[4]

More directly, treating the underactive adrenal problem with low doses of adrenal hormone usually banishes the symptoms of low blood-sugar. I prefer using prescription hydrocortisones such as Cortef instead of the adrenal glandulars available at health food stores. The adrenal content of over-the-counter adrenal glandulars is unknown and varies from batch to batch. Toxicity, or overdosing, is too easy.

TOXICITY OF ADRENAL HORMONES

Adrenal hormones are essential for life. Without them, a person dies. But, as with any hormone, too much can be dangerous. In the early studies using adrenal hormones, the researchers had no idea what dose was normal and what was toxic. When they gave injections of the hormone to patients, the patients' arthritis went away and the patients felt better. However, when they gave a patient many times more than the normal amount, the patient became toxic and died. The researchers were eventually frightened away from adrenal hormones, avoiding their use whenever possible. Medical students were taught to avoid adrenal hormones unless no other treatment choices existed.

The use of adrenal hormones needs to be put into perspective, however. Imagine if the early thyroid researchers had given their patients fifty times the usual dose of thyroid hormone. Thyroid patients would have routinely died of heart attacks. The thyroid researchers, though, were fortunate enough to stumble upon the body's healthy dose early on and to skip negative outcomes. If they had not, people today would not be treated for an underactive thyroid until they displayed symptoms of very advanced thyroid disease (myxedema) or were nearly comatose. Medical science is just beginning to learn that a person can feel horrible and function poorly even with a minimal to moderate hormone deficiency. Waiting for the person to go "off the deep end" of the test's normal scale does not serve any purpose.

Dr. Jeffries has found that as long as the adrenal-hormone level is kept within the normal range, the main toxicity that a patient might experience is a slight upset stomach, due to the body not being used to having the hormone come in through the stomach.[5] Taking the hormone with food usually helps. In addition, some patients gain a few pounds. This is because a low adrenal level can cause a patient's weight to drop below the body's normal "set point," even if that "set point" is high according to society's standards or that person's wishes. However, any weight gain often is more than offset by the weight loss resulting from being able to exercise once again.

Many physicians do not like to prescribe even low doses of adrenal hormone. If your physician does not, have him read Dr. Jeffries' material on the safety of low-dose cortisone.[2,5] Recently, studies have been published about bone loss with low-dose adrenal hormones, but even these studies do not show significant bone loss at the doses that I use.[6] Nonetheless, it is reasonable to take 1,000 milligrams of calcium a day, as well as 400 international units (IU) of vitamin D if your multivitamin does not already contain this amount of vitamin D. Or, include two cups of yogurt with live and active yogurt cultures in your daily diet. After feeling well for six to twelve months, most patients are able to begin slowly decreasing their adrenal-hormone dose, eventually discontinuing the treatment entirely.

If your symptoms started suddenly after a viral infection, if you suffer from hypoglycemia, or if you have recurrent infections that take a long time to resolve, you probably have an underactive adrenal gland. About two-thirds of my severe chronic fatigue patients have an underactive or marginally functioning adrenal gland or a decreased adrenal reserve.[1]

One other item of note is that licorice (real licorice, not the candy that is sold in the United States) and licorice extract can increase adrenal-hormone levels. However, I do not recommend treating with licorice because everybody reacts differently to it and ascertaining just how much it has increased the adrenal-hormone level is difficult. Although I prefer natural products to pharmaceuticals, in this case I am most comfortable with standardized hormones. If the amount of hormone given is within the body's normal range, the body can decide for itself how much of the hormone it wants to use.

The adrenal gland makes many hormones in addition to hydrocortisone. One of these is DHEA. DHEA is often *very* low in CFS patients. Although DHEA's function is not yet fully understood, it appears to be important for good health,[7-9] which makes a low DHEA level worth treating. Some studies suggest that the higher a person's DHEA level is, the longer that person will live and the healthier he or she will be. For many patients, when a low DHEA level is treated, the result is a dramatic boost in energy. I recommend beginning treatment with 5 to 20 milligrams per day of DHEA and slowly working up to what feels like an optimal level to you. In women, I suggest keeping the DHEA-S level at around 150 to 200 micrograms per deciliter, which is the middle of the normal range for a twenty-nine-year-old female. In men, I keep the DHEA-S level between 350 and 500 micrograms per deciliter, which is the normal range for a twenty-nine-year-old male. The low ends of these normal ranges are normal only for people over eighty. If you have side effects such as facial hair or acne, which are uncommon, check your blood level of DHEA-S and decrease your dose back into the normal range. DHEA is available by mail order with a prescription (see Appendix I: Mail Order Sources).

Another important function of the adrenal gland is maintaining blood volume and pressure. Low blood pressure and dehydration are common in CFS patients. Recent research at Johns Hopkins Hospital in Baltimore has suggested that a low dose of a prescription adrenocorticoid such as Florinef can dramatically improve how fatigue patients feel. The researchers suspect that the CFS patient's blood pressure drops precipitously at times and triggers symptoms that can last for weeks.[10] Florinef, which helps the body retain water, can prevent this. Begin with one-quarter of a .1-milligram tablet per day and increase by a quarter tablet every four to seven days until you reach one whole tablet. Note that you may not see any effects for three to six weeks. Drinking plenty of water and getting enough salt and potassium are also helpful.

Hypothyroidism

The thyroid gland, located in the neck area, is the body's gas pedal. It regulates the body's metabolic speed. If the thyroid gland produces insufficient thyroid hormones, the metabolism decreases and the person gains weight. It is not uncommon, in fact, for CFIDS patients to put on 20 to 50 pounds during the first year of their disease. Other symptoms of hypothyroidism include cold intolerance, fatigue, achiness, confusion, and constipation.

The thyroid makes two primary hormones. They are:

- *Thyroxine (T_4)*. T_4 is the storage form of thyroid hormone. The body uses it to make triiodothyronine (T_3), the active form. Most synthetic thyroid medications, such as Synthroid and Levothroid, are pure T_4. These synthetics are fine if your body has the capability to turn them into T_3. Many patients find that their bodies do not.

- *Triiodothyronine (T_3)*. T_3 is the active form of thyroid hormone. Although in some life-threatening illnesses the body appropriately makes less T_3, experience suggests that at times it may not be able to turn T_4 into T_3 when necessary. Most doctors never check T_3 levels. They need to check total or free T_3 levels and directly monitor T_3 function. As just mentioned, the synthetic thyroid medications do not contain T_3. However, the natural thyroid hormones, such as Armour Thyroid, do.

Many years ago, while I was in medical school, physicians were taught to diagnose hypothyroidism, or low thyroid function, by using the newly discovered method of measuring the metabolic rate while the patient ran on a treadmill. Doctors thought that this was a wonderful new test and that they finally had a way to identify patients with underactive thyroids. Doctors congratulated themselves on being so clever. But then a new test came out. The new test measured protein-bound iodide (PBI). When doctors began using the PBI test, they realized, "Oh, we missed diagnosing so many people with a low thyroid, but this new test will now pick up everybody who has a problem." The doctors patted themselves on the back and told all their newly discovered thyroid patients that it turned out that they were not crazy--they just had a low thyroid. The doctors were comfortable that they could now determine with certainty when someone had a thyroid problem.

Then the T_4-level thyroid test was developed and the doctors said, "Oh, that silly old PBI test. It missed so many people with a low thyroid, but this new test will find everyone." Then the T_7-level test came out, and then the thyroid-stimulating hormone (TSH) test. Modern medicine is now into the fourth generation of TSH tests, and with each new test, doctors realize they missed many people with underactive thyroids. You would think that we doctors would finally catch on.

My impression, and the impression of many other physicians, is that the current method of testing still misses *many* people with underactive thyroids. Therefore, doctors must treat the patient, not the blood test. To make matters more difficult, if the thyroid is underactive because the hypothalamus is suppressed, the test may appear to be normal, or even on the high side of normal.[11] (For a more complete discussion of the interpretation of thyroid tests, see Appendix A: For Physicians.)

If you suffer from chronic fatigue plus have achy muscles and joints, heavy periods, constipation, easy weight gain, cold intolerance, dry skin, thin hair, a change in your ankle reflexes called a delayed relaxation of the deep tendon reflex (DTR), or a body temperature that tends to be on the low side of normal, you should consider asking your doctor to prescribe a low dose of thyroid hormone. As long as you do not have underlying angina and you follow up with a blood test to make sure that your thyroid levels are in a safe range, you will find an empiric trial of low-dose thyroid hormone safe and maybe dramatically beneficial.

Some patients have found desiccated thyroid (Armour Thyroid) to be helpful and the synthetic thyroid (Synthroid) not to be. Some have found the opposite. I have found—either through blood testing or according to symptoms—that about 47 percent of my chronic fatigue patients have a low thyroid and that 83 percent of these patients have improved by taking a low dose of thyroid hormone.[1] If you have fibromyalgia and are not treated for an underactive thyroid (even if your blood tests come back normal), your fibromyalgia simply will not resolve. Many physicians who are experts on chronic fatigue agree.[12-14]

Some physicians recommend checking your axilla (armpit) temperature each morning when you first wake up. Before you get out of bed, put a thermometer under your arm and lie quietly for ten minutes. If your temperature is routinely under 97.4°F, consider a trial of thyroid hormone regardless of what your blood test shows.

Low Estrogen, Testosterone, and Oxytocin

Many people going through the change of life develop fatigue or depression. This includes men and women alike. Men and women experiencing a decreased libido also feel fatigued and depressed. Researchers have found that if the estrogen level in females or testosterone level in males is low, a trial replacement of these hormones can bring about dramatic improvement and is therefore worth considering. Some researchers have also wondered if females can have a low testosterone level due to an underactive adrenal gland. Although the ovaries make most of a woman's estrogen and the testicles make most of a man's testosterone, the adrenals make small but significant amounts of both regardless of sex. That females begin with much lower DHEA and testosterone levels than males do may be one factor that increases women's risk of getting CFIDS.

A lot of controversy surrounds who benefits from taking estrogen when going through the change of life. Overall, studies suggest that women who have an increased risk of heart disease (based on high cholesterol, diabetes, family history, and so on), who have osteoporosis, or who have had a hysterectomy will have longer and healthier lives if they take estrogen.[15] If a woman has not had a hysterectomy, she should take progesterone along with the estrogen to prevent uterine cancer. Patients who have been diagnosed with breast cancer should avoid estrogen, as should women whose mother or sister had breast cancer.

If you are a woman who is going through menopause and you prefer not to continue menstruating, you should consider taking estrogen and a decreased dose of progesterone together instead of in cycles. On this regimen, your period may disappear in six to nine months.[16] Some women have found that natural estrogens and progesterones work better and have fewer side effects than the synthetics do. You can use 2.5 to 5 milligrams of the natural estrogen triestrogen daily throughout the month, adding 200 milligrams of progesterone from day one through day fourteen of the month. Keep in mind that 2.5 milligrams of triestrogen equals .625 milligrams of Premarin. Triestrogen and progesterone are both available by mail order with a prescription (see Appendix I).

If you are a man with low testosterone, I recommend a trial of testosterone shots. Testosterone shots have markedly improved the energy level of many men. They also are less likely to trigger cholesterol problems than are testosterone tablets. Although the old testosterone patches were fairly useless, the new testosterone patches (for example, Androderm brand) may work slightly better. Some women may benefit from low doses of oral testosterone.

Drs. Jorge Fletchas and Jay Goldstein, two physicians who do a lot of work with CFS patients, have found that many patients improve through the use of oxytocin. Oxytocin is a hormone produced by the hypothalamus. It is recognized primarily for its function in labor and lactation, but it also appears to be important in the day-to-day performance of the hypothalamus. The hypothalamus, as already discussed, is the master gland of the body.

Dr. Fletchas recommends first bringing the DHEA-S level up to midrange for three months (see page 32) as well as taking 1,500 milligrams each of choline and inositol every day for several weeks before beginning the oxytocin. No blood tests exist for oxytocin deficiency, but Dr. Fletchas feels that patients who are pale and have cold extremities are most likely to benefit from treatment. The doctor advises taking about 10 IU per day. Although oxytocin is best known for its role in stimulating labor, it is also an important neurotransmitter (communication agent) in the brain.[17,18] If the oxytocin treatment is going to help, it should do so in one to two weeks. According to Dr. Fletchas and other experts, 10 IU is the amount of oxytocin that is released by the body during orgasm.[18,19]

Women should note that it is normal for menstruation to

become irregular for the first several months of treatment. This occurs even in women who do not take hormonal treatment, and it resolves on its own.

Other Hormonal Problems

Clinical experience has shown that some patients with diffuse hypothalamic or pituitary disease do not respond to treatment, even when their adrenal hormone, thyroid hormone, oxytocin, estrogen, and testosterone are replaced. Current research suggests that inadequate growth hormone may be an important factor for these patients.[20] Growth hormone (GH) is synthesized and stored in the pituitary gland and assists protein synthesis in the body and bone growth in the limbs. It is also responsible for stimulating DHEA production. Excellent studies recently completed by Drs. William Bennett and Peter Behan, noted CFS-fibromyalgia researchers, show that people with CFS have a significantly diminished GH level. Other studies have shown that low GH levels can be associated with significant fatigue and CFS-like symptoms. The symptoms were shown to improve with treatment.[21-24] In the future, growth hormone may help those few CFIDS patients who do not improve with the current treatment approach. However, treatment with growth hormone is expensive, averaging around $20,000 per year. Fortunately, though, there is a good chance that much of the benefit of GH treatment can be obtained by taking DHEA.

Patients who are lightheaded or drink more water than normal may be low on vasopressin.[25] Vasopressin deficiency can cause low blood pressure and secondary fatigue. Vasopressin, which is also known as the antidiuretic hormone (ADH), is secreted by the pituitary gland and keeps the body from losing too much water by increasing the amount that is reabsorbed by the kidneys. The simplest treatment for a low vasopressin level is to use plenty of salt and water. Some patients find that taking .1 milligram of Florinef along with potassium every day dramatically improves all their symptoms and is worth a six- to eight-week trial. (For a discussion of adrenocorticoids, see page 32.)

The use of prescription adrenocorticoids such as Florinef for fatigue states is still considered experimental. However, they are routinely used for other conditions and are considered fairly safe. Recent research at Johns Hopkins Hospital has shown that Florinef helps neurally mediated hypotension, which is common in CFIDS. Desmopressin, a synthetic derivative of vasopressin that is available as a nasal spray, is rarely helpful.

Prolactin levels are sometimes mildly elevated in CFS patients. Prolactin, another hormone synthesized and stored in the pituitary gland, is best known for stimulating milk production after childbirth. A mildly elevated prolactin level usually has no effect on the patient and may simply reflect hypothalamic injury. To make sure that no pituitary tumor exists, however, I usually order magnetic resonance imaging (MRI) in patients with elevated prolactin levels. The MRI generally shows that everything is normal.

Some physicians have also reported *diabetes mellitus* in the later stages of CFS, although I have not seen this problem in my patients. Dr. Jeffries, interestingly, has found that diabetes often improves through treatment with low-dose cortisol.

As you can see from this chapter, many problems can occur when the body's glands do not function properly. The good news is that most of these problems can be easily treated. In my experience, this has often resulted in dramatic improvement. It is important, though, to treat the *whole* person, not just the hormonal problem.

Important Points

- Underactive adrenals are common in CFS. Treat low or borderline adrenal function with Cortef and/or DHEA (adrenal hormones). If you take Cortef, consider also taking supplemental calcium and vitamin D, or yogurt. If your blood pressure is low, try Florinef (an antidiuretic), increase your water intake, and make sure you consume enough salt and potassium.

- Hypothyroidism is also very common in CFS. Treat low or borderline thyroid function with Synthroid (a synthetic thyroid hormone) or Armour Thyroid (a natural thyroid hormone).

- If you are a woman with an estrogen deficiency or a man or woman with a testosterone deficiency, consider a trial replacement of these hormones.

- Treat an oxytocin deficiency with oxytocin tablets.

- Treat vasopressin deficiency with increased intake of salt, potassium, and water. Add Florinef if the fatigue persists.

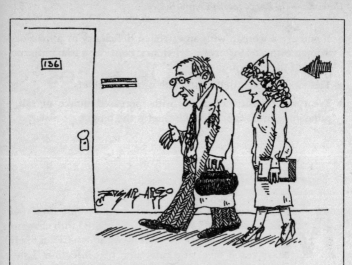

"I'm just an old, country doctor... I don't hold much
with all of this mumbo-jumbo about bacteria."

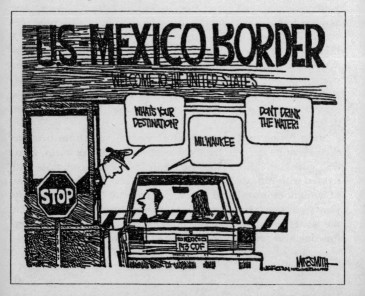

4

When Your Defenses Are Down

Medical science has known for quite some time that chronic fatigue syndrome is associated with changes in the body's immune system. Although CFS is likely triggered by a viral infection, that infection, I suspect, is no longer active in most cases. However, the body acts as if it is. This results in elevated interferon levels.

The body produces interferon to fight a viral infection. When a cancer or hepatitis patient is injected with interferon, the patient becomes achy, fatigued, and brain fogged.[1,2] An underactive adrenal can also cause interferon levels to become elevated.[3] Because of this, it is more accurate to say that the body's immune system is not functioning properly than that it is underactive. Indeed, in many ways, the immune system may be in overdrive and soon exhaust itself. The immune system dysfunctions in many other ways, too, including decreasing the effectiveness of the body's "natural killer" cells, which are an important defense mechanism.[4,5]

Many people suffer recurrent or unusual infections because their immune systems are malfunctioning. Chronic sinus, bladder, prostate, and respiratory infections are common and treated with repeated courses of antibiotics. This large amount of antibiotics introduced into the system can cause a secondary yeast overgrowth because it changes the natural balance between the bacteria and yeast in the bowel. The original immune dysfunction also contributes to the yeast overgrowth. Although it is controversial, a theory held by many physicians is that chronic overgrowth of yeast due to overuse of antibiotics is a potential and strong trigger for chronic fatigue, fibromyalgia, and further immune dysfunction. What makes the theory controversial is that no definitive tests exist to distinguish fungal overgrowth from normal fungal levels. Also, many of the symptoms ascribed to yeast overgrowth can come from other problems, several of which we have already discussed.

CFS patients also frequently have bowel parasite infections. Bowel parasites can cause severe allergic or sensitivity reactions, which in turn can trigger fibromyalgia and fatigue. Often, a patient will finally recover from long-standing and disabling fatigue within a week after beginning treatment for bowel parasites.

Many people are left with disabling fatigue after a bout with infectious Lyme disease or polio. This fatigue also usually responds to the treatments discussed in this book.

Yeast Overgrowth

Everyone's immune system has strong spots as well as weak spots. Some people never get colds but have frequent bouts with athlete's foot or another skin fungal infection. Other people never get fungal infections but tend to get bowel infections. Many people have a diminished ability to fight off fungal infections.

Fungi are very complex organisms. Fungal overgrowth can suppress the host body's immune system. The host body may also develop allergic reactions to components of the yeast. Many physicians feel that yeast overgrowth causes a generalized suppression of the immune system. In other words, once the yeast get the upper hand, they set up a vicious cycle that further suppresses the body's defenses.[6]

As already noted, this theory is controversial. Yeast are normal members of the body's "zoo." They live in balance with bacteria, some of which are helpful and healthy and some of which are detrimental and unhealthy. The problems begin when this harmonious balance shifts and the yeast begin to overgrow. Many things can prompt yeast to overgrow. One of the most prevalent is frequent antibiotic use. When the good bacteria in the bowel are killed off by antibiotics along with the bad bacteria, the yeast no longer have competition and begin to overgrow. The body often is able to rebalance itself after one or several courses of antibiotics, but after repeated or long-term courses—and especially if the body has an underlying immune dysfunction—the yeast can get the upper hand.

Many physicians have also found that sugar stimulates yeast overgrowth. Sugar is food for yeast. Yeast ferment sugar in order to grow and multiply. Yeast overgrowth due to overuse of sugar also seems to cause immune suppression, which facilitates bacterial infections, which require antibiotic use.

A number of very effective methods can be utilized to take care of a yeast problem. Primary among them is to avoid sugar and other sweets. You can enjoy one or two pieces of fruit a day, but you should not consume concentrated sugars such as juices, corn syrup, jellies, or honey. You should stay far away from soft drinks, which have twelve teaspoons of sugar in every twelve ounces. Be prepared to have withdrawal symptoms for about one week when you cut sugar out of your diet. Several excellent books have been written on the yeast controversy and offer additional methods to try. One of the best is *The Yeast Connection and the Woman* by Dr. William Crook.

Many patients have found that acidophilus—that is, milk bacteria, a healthy bacteria for the bowel—helps restore balance in the bowel. Acidophilus is found in yogurt with live and active yogurt cultures. Indeed, a recent study showed that one cup of yogurt a day can markedly diminish the frequency of recurrent vaginal yeast infections.[7] Acidophilus is also available in capsule form.

Nystatin, an antifungal medication, has also been helpful. Unfortunately, many strains of *Candida albicans*, which is the type of yeast that grows in the body, seem to be resistant to nystatin. In addition, nystatin is poorly absorbed, which means that it has little impact on the yeast outside of the bowel. Other antifungal medications, such as Diflucan and Sporanox, seem to be effective systemically—that is, throughout the body—but they have two main drawbacks. First, they are expensive, costing about $450 to $500 for a two-month course. Second, the same as any effective antifungal, they can initially make the symptoms of yeast infection worse.

If the symptoms of the infection are caused by an allergic or sensitivity reaction to the yeast body parts, they may flare when mass quantities of the yeast are suddenly killed off. This happens especially in patients who have severe achiness from the yeast. Because of this reaction, some patients fare better by starting their treatment with acidophilus and a sugar-free diet for a few weeks. I recommend 4 billion IU of acidophilus per day. Next, I have my patients add nystatin in the form of 500,000-IU tablets or powder. I generally recommend beginning with one tablet a day for one to three days and increasing by one tablet every one to three days until two tablets four times a day is reached. Take these eight tablets daily for five to eight months. I add the Diflucan or Sporanox one month after beginning the nystatin. Take 200 milligrams every morning for six weeks. If necessary, take just 100 milligrams per morning for the first three to seven days. If a patient reports any symptoms recurring after stopping the Diflucan or Sporanox, I recommend continuing the medication for an additional six weeks, 200 milligrams a day.

Both Diflucan and Sporanox should be taken with food. If they are taken alone, their absorption is greatly reduced. *Do not use the antihistamine Seldane or Hismanal or the bowel medicine Propulcid with Diflucan or Sporanox.* Also, antacid medications—such as Tagamet, Axid, Zantac, and Pepcid—prevent the proper absorption of Sporanox. At the price per dose, you will want to absorb every last bit of the medication. If you need to be on an antacid medication, use Diflucan instead of Sporanox.

Some patients have also had success using a natural antifungal such as caprylic acid. In addition, many people believe that odorless garlic in capsule or pill form helps combat yeast overgrowth.

I feel that once the yeast has been effectively decreased and kept that way for six to twelve months, it is safe to try to add *small* amounts of sugar back into the diet. If symptoms recur, however, stop the sugar again. Continuing to eat yogurt with live and active acidophilus cultures (unless you are lactose intolerant) or continuing to take acidophilus capsules may also help. Please note that the only kind of acidophilus capsule that is clearly effective against yeast overgrowth is the kind that should be refrigerated. Make sure it was refrigerated in the store and be sure to refrigerate it once you get it home. Otherwise, all you may end up doing is consuming *dead* milk bacteria.

Many books on yeast overgrowth advise readers to avoid all yeast in the diet. This advice is based on the theory that an allergic reaction to yeast is the cause of the problem. The predominant yeast that seems to be involved in yeast over-growth, though, is *Candida albicans*, as already mentioned, al-though I would not be surprised if researchers discovered that other kinds of fungal infections are also involved. The yeast that is found in most foods (except beer and cheese) is not closely related to *Candida*.

In my experience, trying to avoid all yeast in foods results simply in a nutritionally inadequate diet and little benefit. Al-though a few people do appear to have true allergies to the yeast in their food, they number only 2 to 5 percent of patients with suspected yeast overgrowth. These patients may benefit from the more strict diet in Dr. Crook's book. Interestingly, after their adrenal insufficiency and yeast overgrowth are treated, most people find that their allergies and sensitivities to yeast and other food products seem to disappear.

One of the main problems connected with yeast overgrowth is verifying that the condition exists. Some physicians believe that looking for microscopic evidence in stool samples is worth-while. Unfortunately, though, no definitive test has yet been developed to verify yeast overgrowth. Because of this, a physician must base the decision to treat on the patient's medical history and risk factors. Dr. Crook has developed a comprehensive questionnaire to help his readers determine for themselves whether they suffer from yeast overgrowth.[6] If you would like to take this self-test, see Appendix D: Yeast Questionnaire.

The best thing that you can do to combat yeast overgrowth is to try to avoid it in the first place. When you get an infection, begin treating it immediately. Hopefully, you can prevent it from turning into a bacterial infection, which would require an anti-biotic. Ask your doctor what measures you can take before resorting to antibiotics. Many good over-the-counter remedies are available. Your pharmacist is also a wealth of information.

Check your local book store or health food store for books on
natural measures. Your health food store proprietor can also
steer you to appropriate natural remedies. For examples of the
many measures that you can take, see Treating Respiratory
Infections Without Antibiotics, on page 47.

If you find that you must take an antibiotic, all is not lost,
however. You can still lessen the severity of yeast overgrowth by
avoiding sweets and by either taking acidophilus capsules or
eating one cup of yogurt with live and active acidophilus cultures
daily.

If you find yourself with a bladder infection, ask your doctor
to prescribe Macrodantin. Some evidence exists that Macrodantin causes less yeast overgrowth than do other antibiotics.[8] Even
with other antibiotics, most bladder infections are knocked out
in one to three days. About ten ounces of unsweetened cranberry
juice a day or cranberry tablets have also been shown to help
suppress recurrent bladder infections.[9]

Nutritional deficiencies such as low zinc or low selenium may
also decrease resistance to yeast overgrowth.[10,11] A good multivitamin supplement, as recommended in Chapter 2, should take
care of these. This is further evidence that all the factors involved
in CFS are closely interrelated.

Bowel Parasite Infections

Not too long ago, the news focused our attention on Milwaukee
because of repeated outbreaks of an infection by a bowel parasite
called *Cryptosporidium*. A cartoon even made the rounds showing
Mexican tourists being warned not to drink the water in Milwaukee! Although for most people, a *Cryptosporidium* infection resolves
on its own within a week or two, for people with immune suppression, this is not the case. In fact, people with acquired immune
deficiency syndrome (AIDS) are particularly susceptible. Scores of
Milwaukeens died from the *Cryptosporidium* outbreaks.

Unfortunately, in many places throughout the United States,
the water supply is contaminated. Parasites are no longer just a
Third World problem. Doctors frequently see cases of infection
by giardia, amoeba, *Cryptosporidium*, and numerous other bowel
parasites.[12] Parasitic infections can mimic CFS.[13-17]

Treating Respiratory Infections Without Antibiotics

Many people do not realize how many things they can do before resorting to using an antibiotic. For example, if you come down with a respiratory infection, try the following:

- Suck on zinc lozenges five to eight times a day until the infection improves. Make sure that the lozenges have *at least* 10 to 20 milligrams of zinc per lozenge. If they have less, they will not be effective. Zinc lozenges have been shown to speed up recovery from a cold by about 40 percent.
- Take 1,000 milligrams of vitamin C four to eight times a day until the infection improves. Reduce the dosage if diarrhea or gas becomes a problem.
- Drink plenty of water and hot caffeine-free tea.
- If you have flulike symptoms such as fever, chills, achiness, or malaise, take the homeopathic remedy Oscillococcinum. This remedy speeds healing and improves comfort. It is most effective if started early in the infection.
- If you have a sinus infection, try a nasal rinse. Dissolve a half teaspoon of salt in a cup of lukewarm water. Inhale some of the solution about one inch up into your nose, one nostril at a time. Do this either by using a baby nose bulb or an eye dropper while lying down or by sniffing the solution out of the palm of your hand while standing by a sink. Then *gently* blow your nose, being careful not to hurt your ears, and repeat with the other nostril. Repeat with each nostril again until the nose is clear. Rinse your nasal passages at least twice a day until the infection improves. Each rinsing will wash out about 90 percent of the infection and make it much easier for your body to heal.
- Take Tylenol for muscle aches and use Cepacol or Chloraseptic mouthwash for sore throats. Saltwater mixed as described for the nasal rinse also helps sore throats.

- The herb echinacea, which is an immune stimulant, can en-
  hance your body's defenses. Use fifty drops, or about one
  dropperful, of the liquid or 300 to 400 milligrams of the dry
  extract three times a day for up to three weeks at a time. The
  herb goldenseal is also helpful.

In addition to trying the above, check your library or local book
store or health food store for helpful volumes on natural remedies.
Talk to your friends—many people have family remedies that
have been handed down through the generations. Antibiotics are
just one sword in the arsenal of weapons that fight illness.

Most labs miss finding parasites when they do stool testing. I
initially tested for bowel parasites by sending my patients' stool
samples to a respected local lab. The tests kept coming back
negative, so I eventually stopped testing. I now do my own stool
testing. If the test is done properly, it is very time consuming,
taking about five hours per specimen. I do both microscopic and
chemical testing for a variety of parasites. The result is that my
tests now frequently turn out positive. In my experience—and in
that of other physicians, too—when you treat a patient for parasites, the patient's fatigue and achiness improve dramatically.[14–17]
If you would like your stool tested, make sure that the lab
specializes in stool testing and that the sample is a purged
specimen. A purged stool specimen is watery and loose, brought
about by the use of one and a half ounces of the laxative Fleet's
Phospho-Soda. The purpose of the stool purge is to get the best
possible stool sample to check for bowel parasites and yeast. The
laxative washes the organisms off the walls of the intestines so
that they can be detected. The routine random tests done in
almost all standard labs are generally not adequate or reliable.
Recently, I spoke with a gastroenterologist friend who noted that
during a certain bowel exam he had performed, he saw thousands of parasites swimming in the patient's large bowel. He
removed a big glob consisting of nothing but mucus and parasites and sent it off to the major local laboratory just for confirmation of the infection and identification of the parasite. Even

this sample came back negative for parasites. This is why I stress that stool testing must be done at a lab that specializes in parasitology. If such a lab does not exist in your area, you can request stool testing for yeast and parasites to be done at my lab. To order a test kit containing the necessary forms, instructions, and specimen containers, contact me at the address listed in Appendix I: Mail Order Sources. When the testing is completed, my lab will send a copy of the results and recommendations to both you and your physician. Great Smoky Mountain Lab (see Appendix I) also does an excellent job with parasitology.

At this point, no good prescription medication is available for *Cryptosporidium* infections. However, an effective herbal treatment is *Artemisia annua*. For most of my patients, I recommend using 1,000 milligrams three times a day for twenty days. Dr. Leo Galland, a parasite specialist, recommends a form of artemisia called tricyclin for many parasitic infections. He recommends taking two tablets three times a day after meals for six to eight weeks. The cost of this antiparasitic herbal preparation is about $30 for fifty tablets. It is available by mail order, but a prescription is necessary (see Appendix I).

Some fibromyalgia patients often have severe constipation from various causes. The herb turkey rhubarb can be very helpful. Begin by taking two capsules before bedtime. After one to two weeks, add one to two capsules in the morning. Continue this regimen for at least six months, which is how long it takes to retrain the bowel. Turkey rhubarb costs about $15 for one hundred capsules. It is available by mail order (see Appendix I).

FILTER YOUR WATER

Water filters can be very helpful in the fight against parasitic infection. However, not all units are designed to filter out parasites. For a water filter to remove parasites, it must have a submicron solid carbon block filter. A good example is the Multipure filter, which can be purchased by mail order (see Appendix I). Check *Consumer's Digest* and *Consumer's Report* for other good units.

When shopping around for a water filter, request the National Sanitation Foundation (NSF) international listing for the specific unit you are considering. NSF is an independent not-for-profit organization that tests and certifies drinking water treatment products. The unit you buy should meet both NSF Health Effects Standard 53 and NSF Aesthetics Standard 42, with class 1 reduction of chlorine and particulate matter. Any unit that does not meet both of these standards, particularly the health standard, is worthless. To verify that a unit does meet these standards, call the NSF at (313) 769–8010.

In addition to verifying that a water filter meets the NSF standards, ask to see its Product Performance Data Sheet. Many states require that this sheet be given to all prospective customers of drinking water treatment devices.

Ask about the range of contaminants that the unit can reduce under NSF Health Effects Standard 53. Most units certified under Standard 53 list only turbidity and cyst reduction. The number of units that also reduce pesticides, trihalomethanes, lead, and volatile organic chemicals is very small. Make sure that the water filter you are considering can remove the specific contaminants that concern you.

Ask if the unit is licensed in such states as California, Colorado, and Wisconsin. These states have some of the toughest certification procedures in the United States.

Finally, ask about the unit's service cycle, which is stated in gallons of water treated. Find out how often you will need to change the filter and what the replacement filters cost.

As the American water supply becomes more contaminated, parasitic bowel infections will likely become more common. These infections, as well as the overgrowth of yeast or toxic bacteria caused by antibiotic use, contribute to feeling poorly.

As you can see, the body's defenses being down plays a large role in chronic fatigue states. The good news is that by treating the many underlying infections common in CFIDS patients, and by treating any hormonal and nutritional deficiencies, you can bring your immune system back to a healthy state!

Important Points

- An important component of CFS is disordered immune function, which opens the door to repeated infections, repeated treatment with antibiotics, and yeast overgrowth.

- Treat yeast overgrowth by avoiding antibiotics and sweets. Many patients have found nystatin and other antifungal medications, such as Diflucan and Sporanox, to be helpful. Acidophilus (milk bacteria) and natural antifungals such as caprylic acid and garlic are also often useful.

- Bowel parasites are common in CFS patients, whose symptoms often respond dramatically to treatment. However, most labs do not detect parasites through stool testing. To get an accurate test result, use a lab that specializes in stool testing.

- Treat *Cryptosporidium* with *Artemisia annua* or tricyclin (herbal antiparasitics).

- Treat constipation with turkey rhubarb (an herb).

- Prevent parasitic infection by using a water filter.

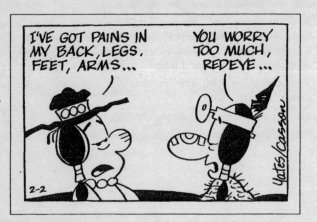

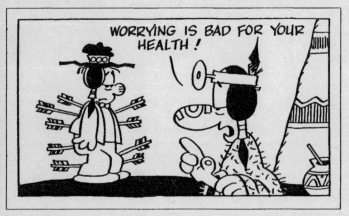

5

Fibromyalgia— The Aching-All-Over Disease

Fibromyalgia, also known as fibrositis, is basically a sleep disorder characterized by many tender knots in the muscles. These tender knots, called tender or trigger points, are a major cause of the achiness that fibromyalgia and CFS patients feel. For most patients, fibromyalgia and CFS are the same illness.

When we sleep, we usually have periods during which we stop moving and go into deep, very restful slumber. Unfortunately, the little muscle knots of fibromyalgia make it uncomfortable to lie in one position for an extended time, causing a return to light sleep. Because of this, fibromyalgia patients do not stay in the deep stages of sleep that recharge their batteries. Although a fibromyalgia patient may sleep twelve hours a night, that patient may not have slept effectively for many years.

Fibromyalgia is a cousin to other muscle diseases, called myofascial pain syndromes. In 1990, the American College of Rheumatology put together a list of criteria for the classification of fibromyalgia (see page 54). The diagnosis of fibromyalgia is made when the patient meets these criteria. To test yourself for fibromyalgia, see Appendix E: Fibromyalgia Information Questionnaire.

Perpetuating Factors of Fibromyalgia

In their excellent 1,300-page review of muscle pain, *Myofascial Pain and Dysfunction: The Trigger Point Manual*, Drs. Janet Travell and David Simons review trigger points and their causes and

Criteria for Fibromyalgia

According to the American College of Rheumatology, patients can be classified as having fibromyalgia if they have:

- *A history of widespread pain.* The patient must be experiencing pain or achiness, steady or intermittent, for at least three months. At times, the pain must have been present:
  - on both the right and left sides of the body.
  - both above and below the waist.
  - midbody—for example, in the neck, midchest, or midback.

- *Pain on pressing at least eleven of the eighteen spots on the body that are known as tender points.* (See Figure 5.1.)

The presence of another clinical disorder, such as arthritis, does not rule out a diagnosis of fibromyalgia.

For more detailed criteria, see Appendix A: For Physicians.

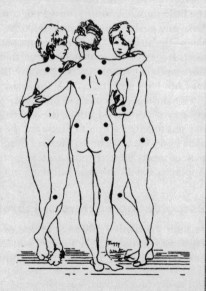

Figure 5.1. Tender point locations on the body.

Criteria and illustration adapted from F. Wolfe, et al., "The American College of Rheumatology 1990 Criteria for the Classification of Fibromyalgia: Report of the Multicenter Criteria Committee," *Arthritis and Rheumatology* 33 (1990): 160–172. Used with permission.

patterns. The authors repeatedly note in their talks and writings that treating the underlying perpetuating factors—that is, the hormonal, nutritional, infectious, and other factors that cause the trigger points to persist—is extremely important. In their chapter on perpetuating factors in *The Trigger Point Manual*, they also address in depth the treatment of major structural problems, such as a short leg or an uneven pelvis (short hemipelvis).[1] It never ceases to amaze me how quickly a case of fibromyalgia can resolve once these underlying problems are treated. The duration of the disease does not seem to impact on how amenable it is to treatment.

Fibromyalgia becomes self-perpetuating as soon as it begins. Even if the underlying trigger, such as a trauma that occurred years before, has resolved, the sleep deprivation of the illness can cause suppression of the hypothalamus.[2] Thyroid and adrenal suppression may also be present, despite the usual blood tests coming back normal.[3] The alteration of sleep then causes fairly marked changes in immune system functioning.[4]

I have found in my practice that fibromyalgia patients tend to recover when all of the major underlying perpetuating factors are treated. An important concept to understand is that fibromyalgia is both a common endpoint for many of the problems we have discussed thus far *and* a cause for these problems. The infections, nutritional deficiencies, and hormonal deficiencies can all, individually and in concert, trigger and perpetuate fibromyalgia. Fibromyalgia can also cause the hormonal and immune dysfunctions and, perhaps by malabsorption, the nutritional deficiencies.

Treatments for Fibromyalgia

A number of treatments currently exist for fibromyalgia that are both necessary and helpful. Among the best are nonaddictive medications that increase deep sleep.[5,6] Many patients improve with just tiny doses of these medications, which is helpful because people with fibromyalgia tend to be very sensitive to medications. I recommend 5 to 50 milligrams of amitriptyline (Elavil), 5 to 20 milligrams of cyclobenzaprine (Flexeril), 25 to 150 milligrams of trazodone (Desyrel), 175 to 350 milligrams of carisoprodol (Soma), and/or 5 to 20 milligrams of zolpidem (Ambien) at bedtime. Often, finding the correct medication is like trying on shoes to see which pair feels the most comfortable.

I tend to prescribe Ambien or Elavil first, unless achiness is a very severe problem, in which case I usually begin with Soma or Flexeril. If anxiety is a significant problem, I might prescribe Desyrel first. Many patients experience next-morning sedation for a while. The degree varies with the medication. Next-morning sedation usually stops being a problem after two to three weeks. Some patients find it helpful to take the medication earlier in the evening—for example, around 7:00—so that the next-day sedation wears off earlier in the morning.

Health food store remedies such as melatonin, passionflower, or a mixture of valerian root and lemon balm improve deep sleep and are less sedating.[7] I tell my patients to try .3 milligram of melatonin, 160 milligrams of passionflower, or 180 to 360 milligrams of valerian root mixed with 90 to 180 milligrams of lemon balm. (To order low-dose melatonin or a valerian root–lemon balm herbal mixture by mail, see Appendix I: Mail Order Sources.) I suspect that many people will find the .3-milligram dose of melatonin to be as effective as and safer than higher doses. Among the prescription medications, Ambien causes the least next-day sedation and in general has the fewest side effects. Unfortunately, it often wears off after five to six hours. Overall, I believe that the sleep medications are more effective than the herbals used alone for fibromyalgia. If the side effects of the medications are a problem, using small doses of several of the medications might help. Another option is using a reduced dose, even one-fourth to one-half of a tablet, *with* the herbals or melatonin. For severe cases of fibromyalgia, especially cases in which the pain is marked, .25 to 2 milligrams of Klonopin (clonazepam) at night can have a dramatic effect. Start with a low dose and work up gradually because Klonopin is initially quite sedating. I use Klonopin as a last resort because it is potentially addictive.

Fibromyalgia patients must also treat their nutritional deficiencies or the illness will persist. Taking a high-level B-complex supplement with minerals, especially magnesium, is critically important. (For a complete discussion of nutritional problems and the supplements I recommend, see Chapter 2.)

Some patients find gentle physical measures to be very helpful. A form of neuromuscular education called Trager, developed by Dr. Milton Trager, has been *very* beneficial for my more severe fibromyalgia patients. Many patients, though, do not need these measures. If your fibromyalgia persists despite the treatments discussed in this book, however, you should consider calling the Trager Institute (see Appendix I) to locate the closest practitioner. The best kinds of Trager practitioners are instructors and tutors. These practitioners have reached a *very* high level of expertise in the technique.

If you decide to see a physical therapist, make sure that you pick someone who is both knowledgeable and gentle. I have seen too many patients made worse by physical therapists who were too rough. With fibromyalgia, gentleness is often much more powerful than roughness. If, however, your body feels like it needs deep work, Rolfing (or structural integration) can be very effective. Rolfing is deep-tissue manipulation and massage. Powerful and *not* gentle, it is designed to relieve and rebalance muscular and emotional tension. To locate a Rolfing practitioner in your area, contact the Rolf Institute (see Appendix I).

Acupuncture is another modality that can be very helpful. Because it approaches health and illness from a very different perspective than traditional medicine does, it can often be very effective in illnesses that resist traditional measures. Many practitioners combine acupuncture with herbal and homeopathic remedies to make their treatments even more effective.

Some fibromyalgia patients find that coenzyme Q_{10}, a nutritional supplement used as an energy source by the muscles, can be helpful. I recommend 30 to 200 milligrams a day. Look for oil-based tablets, which some experts feel are absorbed better. Coenzyme Q_{10} is somewhat expensive but can often be obtained at a discount by mail order (see Appendix I).

Sublingual (under the tongue) nitroglycerin sometimes dramatically eases fibromyalgia pain for three to four hours in about 25 percent of patients. Ask your doctor if you can try a .2-milligram tablet before he or she writes you a prescription. You may get a headache or lightheadedness the first few times you use nitroglycerin, so make sure that you are sitting. The headache usually goes away with Tylenol and time, and often it does not recur. The first one to two doses should tell you if nitroglycerin will work for you. Set aside an eight-hour period each day during which you do not use the medicine so that it remains effective. While you sleep would be perfect.

Some patients use aspirin or ibuprofen for the achiness of fibromyalgia. If it helps, it is worth using. Most often, however, aspirin products are minimally effective and can worsen food sensitivities or ulcers. Most patients find that their bedtime dose of Ambien, Flexeril, Soma, Klonopin, Elavil, or Desyrel is effective without aspirin. If daytime pain relief is needed, Ultram, a new medication, can be very helpful.

Treating structural problems is also critical in fibromyalgia. If one leg is just a quarter- to a half-inch shorter than the other, the entire gait can be thrown off and the muscles put into spasm. If a straight line is drawn through the top of the right and left hipbones, that line should be parallel to the ground when both feet are together. If the hips are not parallel to the ground, the shoulders often are also uneven. For example, if the left hip is higher than the right hip, the left shoulder is often lower than the right shoulder. This is the body's attempt to maintain balance, but it puts a significant strain on the other muscles. Using a small insert called an orthotic in the shoe of the short leg to make the hips the same height can make a world of difference. First, however, see a chiropractor who does a lot of hands-on work, as opposed to one who mainly uses machines. A series of good chiropractic treatments can often balance the hips and resolve the leg-length difference.

If you find that one hip is lower than the other when you sit, try using a butt-lift, a support that goes under the low side to make the hips even. Often, a chiropractor or a physiatrist (physical therapy physician) can be of benefit. Rolfing can also help correct structural problems.

Many patients find that body work also releases suppressed feelings and memories from the muscles. Experience, feel, and embrace these. Your awareness, experience, and release of these feelings is an important part of the healing process.

As you can see, the underlying causes of the disease processes, and indeed the disease processes themselves, are often the same in fibromyalgia and chronic fatigue syndrome. By treating these underlying nutritional, hormonal, and infectious problems, as well as the underlying sleep disorder, most patients improve their fibromyalgia—and many even banish it!

Important Points

- Fibromyalgia is a sleep disorder characterized by multiple tender areas in the muscles. Treat it with medications that increase deep sleep, such as Elavil, Flexeril, Desyrel, Soma, or Ambien. Herbal remedies, such as passionflower or a combination of valerian root and lemon balm, may also help, as can supplemental melatonin (a hormone). Klonopin is useful when pain is severe, but it is potentially addictive.

- Treat nutritional deficiencies with a daily multivitamin that is high in the B vitamins and magnesium, preferably magnesium malate.

- Consider massage or body work, such as Trager or Rolfing.

- Acupuncture is sometimes helpful.

- Coenzyme Q_{10} has helped some patients.

- For extra pain relief, try sublingual nitroglycerin, aspirin, ibuprofen, or Ultram.

- Treat structural problems. Orthotics, chiropractic treatment, or Rolfing can be very helpful.

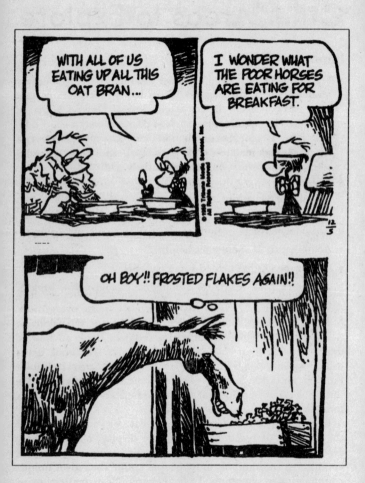

6

Other Areas to Explore

Most patients obtain full resolution of, or at least substantial improvement in, their symptoms with the approaches we have thus far discussed. However, some patients still suffer significant disabilities. Several physicians have found success with treatments that I rarely use. Many of these treatments are worth exploring. In addition, two areas remain that I hold in high regard and stress with all my patients—exercise and being gentle with yourself.

Food Allergies

I have found that most of my patients' food and other sensitivities resolve when I treat their underlying yeast overgrowth, parasitic infections, or underactive adrenal glands. Occasionally, though, I steer a patient toward a self-help book on how to determine and treat your own food allergies. The book that I usually recommend is *How to Control Your Food Allergies* by Robert Forman, Ph.D (see Appendix C: Recommended Reading). Sadly, this book is out of print, but you might be able to find it at your local library or in a used book store.

Food allergies are often hard to isolate or verify because of the diversity of reactions that people display. Many of these reactions are extremely subtle or are also symptoms of other conditions. In addition, most people suffer their own unique combination of symptoms. To further complicate matters, many people are sensitive to food additives, which are listed on food

labels under a variety of names or are present as integral parts
of other additives. A prime example is monosodium glutamate
(MSG). For a discussion of the variety of allergic reactions that
MSG has caused in consumers and a list of the foods and food
additives that generally contain it, see Sensitivity Reactions to
Monosodium Glutamate, on page 64.

Dr. Jeffrey Bland, a well-known nutritional biochemist, has a
food product that can be used with an elimination diet to
determine food allergies. The product is a powder that supplies
all the necessary nutrients from very low allergy sources, such as
rice. During the initial seven to ten days of the elimination diet,
it allows you to avoid all "allergic foods." If your symptoms
resolve during this time span, you are justified in suspecting that
you have food allergies. You can then begin reintroducing the
different foods as described below to determine exactly which
ones are problems for you. Although Dr. Bland's food product
costs about $300, it is the most effective way that I have found
to determine food sensitivities. However, do not use this approach if you have very severe CFS—for example, if you are
bedridden—because you need to strengthen your body as much
as possible before you go through the withdrawal phase. For
more information on Dr. Bland's powder, contact Metagenics
(see Appendix I: Mail Order Sources).

Unfortunately, I have found the radioallergosorbent test
(RAST) and cytotoxic test, two blood tests used to detect food
allergies, to not be very helpful. They are more expensive than
Dr. Forman's and Dr. Bland's approaches and leave people with
the incorrect belief that they are sensitive to everything. I have
found that these tests are better at making people crazy than at
distinguishing true allergies. I use a blood test that screens for
ten common foods and is more likely to give a false negative than
a false positive result. However, the best approach that I have
found for determining what food allergies, if any, are present is
the elimination diet.

In an elimination diet, the most common problem foods are
eliminated from the diet for two weeks. The foods that seem to
cause problems for the most people are milk, wheat, eggs, citrus,
monosodium glutamate (MSG), sugar, alcohol, chocolate, and
coffee. People with food allergies usually go through withdrawal

when they cut out the foods to which they are allergic. They feel worse for the first seven to ten days. But once they get over the hump, they often feel dramatically better. The eliminated food groups are then reintroduced, one every few days, to isolate the specific problem foods. These problem foods are left out of the diet for a few months and then are slowly reintroduced, since the sensitivity often will have decreased. Once reintroduced, the problem foods are initially used only every three to seven days to see how they are tolerated.

Many physicians who practice what is called clinical ecology use sublingual neutralization, among other approaches, and are very skilled at treating food allergies. Although I am not familiar with these approaches and although they are controversial, I have seen them work wonders for many patients.

Chemical Sensitivity

Clinical ecologists can be especially helpful for people who have multiple chemical sensitivity syndrome. I believe that this syndrome is a subset of chronic fatigue syndrome. In multiple chemical sensitivity syndrome, the body has given up and is reactive to almost everything in the environment.

Many CFS patients have multiple allergies and sensitivities to environmental chemicals and medications. However, while this is common, it is *not* multiple chemical sensitivity syndrome.

Patients with multiple chemical sensitivity syndrome cannot live in a normal house because they can become deathly ill if a new carpet is put in, if the walls are painted or wallpapered, or if pesticide is sprayed. They can become ill just from washing the dishes or reading a book. They can react negatively to any or all of the thousands of chemicals with which we normally come in contact in our day-to-day lives.[1-3] For patients who have this very extreme problem, I recommend an excellent book by Sherry Rogers, M.D., entitled *Tired or Toxic* (see Appendix C).

Rare Infections

There is also a subset of patients who seem to be infected by agents that we have not yet been able to culture. I have learned

Sensitivity Reactions to Monosodium Glutamate

Monosodium glutamate (MSG) is a naturally occurring form of glutamic acid, an amino acid that is extracted from certain vegetables and grains. It is popular among Asian cooks for adding "zing" to dishes, but experts disagree on how it does this. What the experts no longer disagree on, however, is that MSG also produces a variety of sensitivity reactions in people. This sensitivity to MSG is called the Chinese restaurant syndrome.

People who react to MSG are really reacting to the *free* glutamic acid that is present in foods as a result of processing. MSG-sensitive people generally do not react to *bound* glutamic acid, which is found in protein, or to free glutamic acid that is present in unadulterated, unfermented food. Why some people react, and why others do not, is not known. Also unknown is whether MSG causes the condition underlying the reaction or simply aggravates an already-existing condition.

The symptoms of MSG reaction, according to the National Organization Mobilized to Stop Glutamate (NOMSG) and the Truth in Labeling Campaign (TLC), "although seemingly dissimilar, are no more diverse than the reactions found as side effects of certain neurological drugs." Among the symptoms they list are the following:

- *Cardiac.* Arrhythmias; extreme drop in blood pressure; rapid heartbeat (tachycardia); angina.
- *Circulatory.* Swelling.
- *Muscular.* Flulike achiness; joint pain; stiffness.
- *Neurological.* Depression; dizziness, lightheadedness, loss of balance; disorientation, mental confusion; anxiety, panic attacks; hyperactivity, behavioral problems in children; lethargy, sleepiness, insomnia; migraine headache; numbness, paralysis; seizures; slurred speech.
- *Gastrointestinal.* Diarrhea; nausea, vomiting; stomach cramps; irritable bowel; bloating.

- *Respiratory.* Asthma, shortness of breath; chest pain, tightness; runny nose, swelling.
- *Skin.* Hives, rash; mouth lesions; temporary tightness or partial paralysis (numbness or tingling) of the skin; flushing; extreme dryness of the mouth.
- *Urological.* Swelling of the prostate; nocturia.
- *Visual.* Blurred vision; difficulty focusing.

If you are sensitive to MSG, make sure that you carefully read the labels on all the food products you consider purchasing. While often listed as "MSG" or "monosodium glutamate," MSG is also often hidden, whether intentionally or unintentionally.

The following foods and additives contain enough MSG to be known as common MSG-reaction triggers:

- Glutamate
- Monopotassium glutamate
- Glutamic acid
- Calcium caseinate
- Sodium caseinate
- Gelatin

- Textured protein
- Hydrolyzed protein
- Yeast extract
- Yeast food
- Autolyzed yeast
- Yeast nutrient

According to NOMSG and TLC, the food items below *often* contain MSG or create it during processing:

- Malt extract
- Malt flavoring
- Barley malt
- Bouillon
- Stock
- Broth
- Carrageanan
- Maltodextrin
- Whey protein
- Whey protein isolate
- Whey protein concentrate
- Pectin

- Protease enzymes
- Enzymes
- Protease
- Flavors and flavorings
- Natural flavors and flavorings
- Natural pork flavoring
- Natural beef flavoring
- Natural chicken flavoring
- Seasonings
- Soy sauce
- Soy sauce extract

- Soy protein
- Soy protein isolate
- Soy protein concentrate
- Anything that is "protein fortified"
- Anything that is "enzyme modified"
- Anything that is "ultra-pasteurized"
- Anything that is "fermented"

In addition, disodium quanylate and disodium inosinate work synergistically with MSG and probably would not be present in a product if MSG were not also used. Low-fat milk products often include milk solids that contain MSG. Nonfood products can also cause problems. Binders and fillers for medications, nutrients, and supplements, both prescription and nonprescription; enteral feeding materials; and some intravenous fluids contain MSG. Soaps, shampoos, hair conditioners, and cosmetics have also caused MSG-type reactions, usually to ingredients that are hydrolyzed or found in amino acids.

People who are MSG sensitive should also try to avoid aspartame, which is sold under the brand name Nutrasweet. The culprit is the aspartic acid in aspartame. Aspartame, as well as MSG, is often found in drinks, candy, and chewing gum. Additionally, aspartame is found in some medications, including children's medications.

For more information on MSG and MSG sensitivity, contact the National Organization Mobilized to Stop Glutamate, P.O. Box 367, Santa Fe, New Mexico 37504, telephone (800) BEAT–MSG; or the Truth in Labeling Campaign, P.O. Box 2532, Darien, Illinois 60561, telephone (312) 643–9393.

from several microbiologists that one agent is especially suspect. Called a mycoplasma, this infectious agent belongs to a group of parasitic microorganisms that do not have rigid cell walls and therefore display numerous forms. It is midway between a bacteria and a larger parasite. The specific mycoplasma suspected of causing problems for CFS patients is the *Mycoplasma incognitus,* or *Mycoplasma fermentans.* Some patients find short-term relief from their chronic fatigue when they take tetracycline for an infection. These patients, I believe, are at high risk for having an unrecognized infection such as this from mycoplasma. This mycoplasma, unfortunately, is resistant to erythromycin.

Doctors who are familiar with the problems caused by yeast overgrowth are very reluctant to prescribe tetracycline, a major player in yeast overgrowth and chronic fatigue states, especially in people who take it for many years for acne. Despite this, if you have found in the past that you feel better after taking tetracycline, or if you have recurrent lung congestion or frequent fevers above 100°F, you should consider a trial of doxycycline, which is a type of tetracycline. I recommend taking 100 milligrams twice a day for three weeks. If your symptoms improve noticeably, mycoplasma may be playing a role in your illness. If your symptoms recur after definite improvement, especially if you have been treating the other problems noted in this book, you should take repeated courses of doxycycline for one to two months at a time until your problem is finally eliminated. However, please note that while you take the doxycycline, you should also take the precautions against yeast overgrowth that are discussed in Chapter 4.

Nasal Congestion and Sinusitis

If you enjoy relief from your chronic fatigue whenever you take tetracycline and if mycoplasma does not seem to be your problem, you may have chronic sinusitis. Dr. Alexander C. Chester III, a physician practicing in Washington, D.C., has been a strong advocate of checking for nasal congestion and sinusitis as a cause of chronic fatigue. He has found that many patients improve significantly by observing a regimen to combat sinusitis. This includes patients who never even suspected that they had nasal problems.[4] Fatigue from nasal problems used to be more recognized in medicine. Its importance is being rediscovered.

The treatment trial that Dr. Chester recommends for nasal congestion and sinusitis includes the following:

- Take 500 milligrams of Keflex four times a day for one week. If you do not see any improvement in your symptoms, take 100 milligrams of doxycycline twice a day for one week. Both Keflex and doxycycline are prescription antibiotics.

- Use Xylometazoline .1-percent nasal spray three times a day for three days. Xylometazoline is a prescription nasal spray.

- Take 60 milligrams of Sudafed four times a day or 120 milligrams of sustained-release Sudafed twice a day for two weeks. Note that Sudafed causes shakiness or palpitations in some people. Sudafed is an over-the-counter decongestant.

- Inhale steam for twenty minutes three times a day for two weeks to open your nasal passages. To do this, boil water in a pot on the stove or fill your bathroom sink with steaming water. Then lean over the water, with a towel draped over your head, and inhale the steam. Be careful not to burn yourself. Better yet, use a nasal steamer (see Appendix I).

- Sleep at least eight hours a night.

- Do not consume any beer, wine, or milk products.

I also recommend following the regimen for respiratory infections described on page 47. If you find your sinus symptoms improving from these regimens, you should consider using a cortisone nasal spray such as Vancenase to maintain the effect. Sometimes, nasal or sinus surgery is needed. For patients with chronic sinusitis, I strongly recommend the book *Sinus Survival* by Robert S. Ivker (see Appendix C).

Sleep Apnea, Restless Legs, and Similar Disorders

Sleep apnea, a condition in which breathing stops intermittently at night, often causes poor sleep and fatigue. It is usually, but not always, associated with overweight and snoring.[5] It is diagnosed by having the patient spend the night being monitored in a sleep lab. Home testing is now also available.

Restless leg syndrome is a condition in which the legs are jumpy during sleep. It also is an important cause of poor sleep and will be picked up during a sleep study.[6]

Grinding the teeth during sleep is a condition called bruxism. It can cause headaches and a sore jaw.

The sleep lab should be able to guide you toward treatment for all of these problems. For bruxism, all you may need is a mouth guard, which is available from your dentist. A daily dose of 600 IU of vitamin E or supplemental iron for six weeks or Sinemet (carbidopa-levodopa), Klonopin, or Neurontin (gabapentin) often decreases restless leg syndrome. For more information on restless legs, send a self-addressed stamped envelope to the Restless Leg Foundation (see Appendix I). For more information on sleep apnea, try to find a copy of the May 1993 issue of the *American Journal of Medicine*. It contains an excellent article by K. P. May, S. G. West, and others entitled "Sleep Apnea in Male Patients With Fibromyalgia."

People who snore loudly (or their spouses!) can wake up exhausted from the snoring. This includes people who do *not* have sleep apnea. Many snorers have found relief using a product called Breathe Right. Available in many pharmacies, these nasal strips can also be purchased by mail (see Appendix I). A new procedure called laser uvuloplasty has been used successfully to eliminate loud snoring. Your otolaryngologist (ear, nose, and throat physician) can either do this procedure or refer you to someone who can.

Seasonal Affective Disorder

If your fatigue is a problem mainly from October to May, is less pronounced on sunny days, and is associated with increased sleep, weight gain, and carbohydrate craving during the winter, you may suffer from sunlight deprivation.[7,8] This malady is known as seasonal affective disorder (SAD), or the winter blues.

SAD is treatable with a light box, which is available by mail order (see Appendix I). Use a 10,000-lux box positioned at a forty-five-degree angle in relation to your face and about eighteen inches away. Spend thirty to forty-five minutes in front of the box every morning from September through May. Add a half hour at night if necessary. Experiment to find the best times of the day and session lengths for you. You do not have to sit still in front of the box but can do table work such as reading, writing, or cutting vegetables.

If you have trouble waking up in the morning, attach a bright (about 250 luxes) bedside lamp to a timer and program it to turn on two hours before your alarm is set to go off. Portable light visors are also currently being tested and are available by mail order (see Appendix I). Most patients find that it takes one to six weeks to see any results.

Serotonin deficiency has also been put forward as a possible cause of SAD. Serotonin is a brain-message transmitter that is connected in particular with the process of sleep. Medications that raise the serotonin level, such as Prozac and fenfluramine, have been shown to be effective against SAD.[9,10]

Medications

Many medications have fatigue as a side effect. If you are on a medication and your fatigue has been worse since you started taking it, talk to your physician about alternative measures or about just stopping it.

Interestingly, a blood pressure raising enzyme called angiotensin converting enzyme (ACE) has been found to be elevated in CFS patients.[11] Despite this, blood pressure may still be low, due to, for example, an underactive adrenal. According to some physicians, CFS symptoms have improved in a few patients who were given ACE inhibitors, such as Accupril, for their hypertension. Other studies have shown that some CFS patients improved with Nimotop (nimodipine) or Calan, calcium-channel blockers that relax the blood vessels to allow more blood and oxygen to get to the heart.[12,13] If your blood pressure is high, you might consider a trial of Nimotop, followed by a trial of Calan and then a trial of Accupril. Try each one for two weeks to see which feels the best to you.

Also Worth Trying

Some patients benefit from taking evening primrose oil plus fish oil. I recommend two 500-milligram capsules of evening primrose oil four times a day and 1,000 milligrams of fish oil once a day. Try to find Efamol or Linus Pauling Brand primrose oil and MaxEPA fish oil. You should begin seeing effects in about three months. When you do, you can experiment with lowering the doses.

Researchers are currently studying high-dose intravenous

gamma globulin and ampligen, both of which are immune-function enhancers. These treatments cost *many* thousands of dollars per year, and I do not think that most patients need them. I do find, though, that weekly intramuscular injections of 4 cubic centimeters (cc) of gamma globulin (Gammar) for four weeks sometimes help patients with recurrent infections. These shots, luckily, are not expensive.

Kutapressin, a liver extract, has also helped patients with severe recurrent infections. The normal dose is 2 cc given intramuscularly every day for three weeks. After the third week, the shots are generally decreased by one a week every one to three weeks until three shots are given per week. It takes three to four weeks to see any effect.

Some patients have found magnesium-potassium aspartate to be very helpful in improving their energy. The aspartate is important to the cells' energy cycle. The dose is 1 gram twice a day. Most patients see an effect within two weeks, at which time they can often reduce their dose.[14]

Magnesium sulphate injected intramuscularly often helps CFS patients, especially those whose achiness is severe but who get diarrhea from oral magnesium. A good dose is 2 grams once a week for four weeks. Magnesium sulphate administered this way is inexpensive, but it can be a "pain in the butt." To combat this problem, I like to add a small amount of Novocain to the shot. Some physicians reduce the magnesium and add the B vitamins, including B_{12}, and calcium. Called a Myers cocktail, this combination, given intravenously, has produced significant benefits, especially in patients whose main problem was achiness, asthma, or migraine.

Coenzyme Q_{10} sometimes helps CFS patients and is just moderately expensive. The recommended dose is 25 to 50 milligrams three to four times a day or a 100-milligram sublingual tablet once or twice a day. Coenzyme Q_{10} can be purchased at a discount by mail order (see Appendix I).

Dr. Jay Goldstein, a well-known researcher working on brain chemistry and CFS, has come up with a long list of recommended treatments that may be helpful. Because the agents he uses act directly on the disordered blood flow in the brain, Dr. Goldstein finds that patients generally know what effect each medication will have within one hour—and even within minutes for some agents. Because the medications that are most likely to be effective from among those on his list are nitroglycerin and Nimotop, I give my patients one-fourth of a .2-milligram nitroglycerin tablet under the tongue and have them wait ten minutes (headache and dizziness are common with the first few doses). If the patient feels better, I prescribe nitroglycerin. I then give my patients 30 milligrams of Nimotop and tell them to wait for one hour. If a patient notes a marked improvement, I prescribe this medication. My usual dose is one tablet one to three times a day. Nimotop, which is used for subarachnoid hemorrhages, or brain bleeds, is usually well tolerated. However, it is also expensive, costing about $3 per tablet. For a complete discussion of all of Dr. Goldstein's treatments, read his book *Betrayal by the Brain* (see Appendix C).

Exercise

Exercise is very important for your sense of well-being. Fibromyalgia patients often find that when they exercise, they feel exhausted the next day. Because of this, they begin a vicious cycle in which they feel that they are unable to exercise, they do not exercise, they become further deconditioned from the lack of exercise, and they feel even more so that they cannot exercise. The good news is that as you treat your CFS problems, your post-exercise exhaustion will change to a "good tired" for a couple of hours after exercising and then to a good feeling the next day.

As your health starts to improve, slowly add exercise to your regime. Begin with something gentle, such as walking or swimming. If you feel exhausted the next day, you probably pushed too hard and should take it easier the next time. Soon, you will find your ability and stamina normalizing. Give yourself time to *slowly* build up, though. You may be severely deconditioned from years of not exercising.

I recommend walking as your primary exercise during the initial stages of your recovery. Walking conditions the heart and muscles and is easy on the joints and ligaments. When you walk outdoors, you can also enjoy the fresh air. Although getting fresh air may seem like a silly point, it is important. Fresh air is good for the lungs and clears the mind. Cold wind, however, causes fibromyalgia symptoms to flare. When the weather is chilly, walk around your local mall. Some malls even host walking clubs. Or, use a stationary bicycle or a NordicTrack-type machine.

Many CFS patients feel a sense of powerlessness and an inability to defend themselves. Although the idea of practicing a martial art may seem impossible right now, you may be pleasantly surprised at your ability when your symptoms resolve. Research the different martial arts that are currently popular and check your Yellow Pages for the closest training center.

Be Gentle With Yourself

People who develop severe chronic fatigue states are often type-A individuals who were overachievers before becoming ill. As they begin to recover, they tend to want to make up for lost time by trying to get everything done that they could not finish while ill. *Do not do this!*

When you first begin recovering, you should reserve the energy that is slowly returning for activities that make you feel good. Most of the things that you have left undone can remain undone. Many probably do not ever need to be done.

As you start feeling better, take your time adding new activities and returning fulfilling old ones to your life. Do just those things that you really want to do. Do not go "shoulding" (should do this, should do that) on yourself.

Although you likely view your illness as an enemy, you should let it become your ally. Many people with CFIDS were caught in what my wife—who I feel knows much more about this illness than I do—calls role entrapment. Role-entrapped people were taught that they have to be the perfect spouse or the perfect parent or the perfect employee. The superwoman complex is a good example. CFIDS can be your body's way of getting out of the roles in which you are trapped. Most of us have so bought into society's expectations of us that we have taken them on as our own. What we fail to recognize is that because of its tremendous rate of acceleration, our current society is an aberration. There has been no other stable society during the last three thousand–plus years, nor are there many others presently on the planet, in which "normal" change occurred so rapidly. Despite all our modern conveniences and laborsaving devices, which were supposed to give us more free time, most people find that they are running ever faster. Where one parent used to be home to take care of the children while the other parent worked, both—if you are lucky enough to have both parents in the same household—now often must work to maintain the family's standard of living.

Because our whole society is trapped in roles, this chaos may seem normal. *It is not.* It is abnormal. Although some people thrive on it, more people every day are becoming burned out. I suspect that the physical processes that make up CFS and fibromyalgia are manifestations of this—and that we are just beginning to see the tip of the iceberg.

As you get well, you will need to reclaim your own natural speed and pace of life. This may mean a somewhat lower standard of living, but you may have been living with that for several years now anyway. On the plus side, it may also mean that your children will have an improved parent and that your life will be more fulfilling. Many people live their lives like hamsters running faster and faster on the exercise wheels in their cages. Give yourself permission to step off the wheel!

Important Points

- Check for food allergies, then temporarily remove the suspect foods from your diet.
- See a clinical ecologist if you have chemical sensitivities that are severe.
- Treat nasal congestion or sinusitis with Keflex or doxycycline (antibiotics), Xylometazoline (a nasal spray), Sudafed (a decongestant), steam, and sleep.
- Consider testing and treatment for sleep apnea, restless leg syndrome, bruxism, or snoring.
- Treat seasonal affective disorder with a light box or a medication that raises the serotonin level, such as Prozac or fenfluramine.

- Ask your doctor for alternatives to medications that have fatigue as a side effect.

- Treat high blood pressure with Nimotop, Calan, or Accupril.

- Patients have also benefited from evening primrose oil, fish oil, gamma globulin shots, kutapressin shots, magnesium-potassium aspartate, magnesium sulphate shots, coenzyme Q_{10}, and a variety of treatments developed by Dr. Jay Goldstein including sublingual nitroglycerin and Nimotop.

- When you can, begin an exercise program. Walking or swimming are excellent for beginners.

- Get plenty of fresh air.

- Do not try to make up for lost time as you start to feel better.

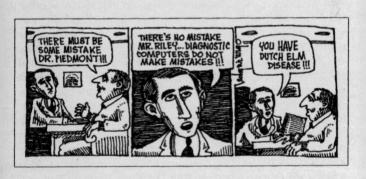

7

Am I Crazy?

In medicine, we have a bad habit. If a doctor cannot figure out what is wrong with a patient, the doctor brands that patient a turkey. Imagine calling an electrician because your lights do not work. The electrician checks all your wiring and says, "You're crazy. There's nothing wrong with your lights." You flip the switches and they still do not work, but the electrician just says, "I've looked. There's no problem here," and walks out the door. This is analogous to what many CFS patients experience. I apologize for the medical profession's calling you crazy just because we cannot determine the cause of your problem. It is inappropriate and cruel.

What you have is a very real and physical illness. And, like most other physical processes—such as diabetes, heart disease, cancer, and ulcers—it has an associated psychological component. As is true for any disease, when you treat the physical component, you must also treat the underlying psychological issues. If you do not, the disease will simply manifest itself in another way.

It might also help you to understand that you may sometimes mistake uncomfortable feelings such as disappointment or sadness for fatigue. Try to be aware of when you do this. There is no such thing as an inappropriate feeling. You have the right to feel whatever you feel.

Does this mean that you are crazy? No. It simply means that, like all human beings, you have emotional issues to deal with as part of your growth process. In my practice, I frequently see CFS patients who seem to be "caught on the horns of a dilemma" emotionally. These patients find themselves in situations in which they are unable to make a choice between two or more alternatives—for example, between working and having children, or between staying with or leaving their spouse. These conflicts come in an infinite variety. Defending yourself against *acknowledging* a conflict can sap your energy.

Unfortunately, some patients become so frustrated by being told their CFS is "all in their head" that they are in a Catch-22. They feel that if they acknowledge that they also have emotional issues (the way everyone does), they are validating the doctors who say that their illness is all emotional. Give yourself permission to be human. You are no more and no less crazy than anyone else.

In my experience, when patients start to feel better physically, they find it easier to deal with their emotional issues. The issues are often holdovers from the past and are now easier to resolve. Actually, however, you do not have to resolve every conflict. If you have something that you cannot settle at your current level of growth, you might find it helpful to simply hold it in your awareness instead of suppressing it. Tell yourself, "Yes, I have these two areas that are in conflict and I cannot reconcile them now." The tension of holding those opposites and the conflict in your awareness will result in psychological growth, the same way that exercising helps a muscle to grow. Many people find that after a while, a solution comes from a new perspective.

A large percentage of CFS patients are type-A overachievers, as discussed in Chapter 6, who were driven by low self-esteem as children.[1] In the first part of their lives, these patients needed to overachieve for their growth and self-image. Although not the preferred method, CFS helps them slow down long enough to reclaim themselves. For many, a period of deep rest is essential. The illness actually serves many patients well. Part of getting well is "lightening up." The old Zen image of worry being an old man carrying a load of feathers that he thinks are rocks often fits perfectly. Many of the worries we carry around sort themselves out as soon as we let go of them. Although things may not always work out the way we would like them to (CFS patients are often "control freaks"), they usually work out for the best. Because of this, it helps to have (or reclaim) a sense of humor.

I am a firm believer in psychological counseling. Counseling is helpful to anybody who is growing. People who are emotionally or intellectually brain-dead and living by a "social cookbook" instead of thinking for themselves may never need counseling. People who are growing, however, frequently come across areas that are difficult and with which it is usual and natural to need help.

Although many CFS patients feel depressed because of their illness, only a small minority have depression as the cause of their fatigue.[2,3] The depression caused by CFS is often simply frustration. Fatigue patients usually have a lot of interests and are frustrated by their lack of energy. If a patient has depression causing fatigue, that patient probably has few interests. The stress of CFS can itself cause depression. When combined with other treatments, the new antidepressants—such as Zoloft, Prozac, Paxil, Serzone, and Effexor—often act as energizers even in the absence of depression. If you use one of these medications, start with a low dose—for example, 10 milligrams of Paxil—and slowly raise it as needed. It takes six weeks to see the full effect. If the effect decreases over time, take Buspar, an antianxiety agent, or increase the antidepressant dose to restore the effectiveness. Although in many ways, depression and CFS are opposites—for example, cortisol levels are high in depression and low in CFS—low serotonin levels are seen in both diseases. Zoloft, Prozac, Paxil, Serzone, and Effexor raise serotonin levels, even when depression is not a factor.

Whether or not you are depressed, you should find some type of therapist for emotional support and guidance. Be careful who you choose, however. Many therapists have never dealt with their own problems and simply work out their personal conflicts and issues on their patients. Others have worked through their issues and are excellent with patients. Talk to your friends and relatives to find somebody who is good. Your physician is an excellent resource. There are many excellent approaches, but my own personal bias is for a therapist who takes a Transpersonal Psychology or Jungian approach. I have found one physician, Brugh Joy, M.D., to be extraordinarily skilled at helping people to understand their deep psyches.

Dr. Joy runs workshops in the Arizona mountains. I cannot recommend these workshops too strongly. They demand a lot of work, are somewhat expensive (although very reasonable for what they give in return), and last approximately twelve days each. They are more effective than a year of regular counseling. For beginners, I recommend the Foundation workshop. Do not attend Dr. Joy's workshops for the purpose of treating your chronic fatigue, however. Instead, go for the goal of learning to accept and understand more fully who you really are. For more information on Dr. Joy's workshops, call Brugh Joy, Inc. (see Appendix I: Mail Order Sources).

By using your chronic fatigue as a springboard for personal growth, you can find your CFS turning into a blessing. I found this to be the case for me. My CFS gave me a firsthand understanding of the problem and a powerful incentive to learn how to overcome it. It also has led me into wonderful areas of growth.

Important Points

- CFS and fibromyalgia are physical processes with physical causes. However, the same as other illnesses, they have psychological components, which must also be treated.

- CFS patients both with and without depression have been helped by the new generation of antidepressants, such as Zoloft, Prozac, Paxil, Serzone, and Effexor.

- Consider therapy for emotional support and guidance.

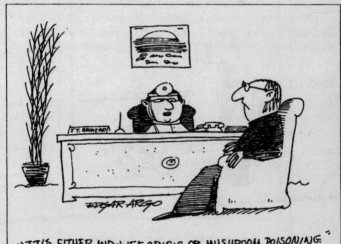

"IT'S EITHER MID-LIFE CRISIS OR MUSHROOM POISONING."

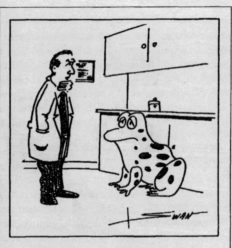

"You must realize there's a great deal modern medical science doesn't understand about curses."

8

Finding a Physician

There are many approaches that you can take to find a physician to help you with your illness. The best place to begin is with your family physician. Although most physicians are too busy to read this whole book, your physician may be willing to read Appendix A: For Physicians and to run the lab tests listed on page 108. If Appendix A stimulates your physician's interest, he or she may then read the whole book. Even if your physician is unwilling to read any of the book, you can ask him or her to run the lab tests and to give you the results to interpret yourself using the test-result explanations on page 109. You can then talk to your physician about trying the necessary treatments. Or, you can ask your physician to allow my lab to run or interpret the tests and to make treatment recommendations (see Appendix I: Mail Order Sources). With my recommendations in hand, your physician may feel more comfortable treating you. Except for the stool tests, though, all the tests can be effectively run in any lab and interpreted by any physician who takes the time to read and follow Appendix A.

In your search for a caretaker, you will discover that physicians tend to fall into three categories:

1. *Simply not interested.* Try another physician.
2. *Skeptical but willing to explore new possibilities.* Offer this physician a copy of Appendix A, as discussed above, or the whole book, if he or she prefers. Be persistent, yet gracious, in encouraging the physician to give the treatments a try. Most

of the treatments are very benign if used in the ways that I
recommend. Although the physician initially may be uncomfortable with using Cortef or DHEA, encourage him or
her to give you a trial prescription. Current evidence suggests that both are reasonably safe in the dosages that I
suggest. I was also uncomfortable with Cortef until I read
the studies and the book on it. (For a complete discussion
of cortisol and my reference sources, see page 27. For a
complete discussion of DHEA and my reference sources,
see page 32.)

3. *Willing to work with you.* Wonderful. You can concentrate
   on getting well rather than on convincing your physician
   to treat you.

If your physician is simply not interested in learning about CFS
or if he or she is skeptical though open but you want someone who
is completely willing, check Appendix H: Physicians Specializing in
Chronic Fatigue Syndrome. Also try the Chronic Fatigue and
Immune Dysfunction Syndrome Association of America, listed in
Appendix G: Patient Support Groups, and the American Holistic
Medical Association and the American College for Advancement
of Medicine, both listed in Appendix H. I *strongly* recommend
joining the Chronic Fatigue and Immune Dysfunction Syndrome
Association of America and the Fibromyalgia Network. These are
two of the best patient support groups I have ever come across.
They can put you in touch with your local support groups, which
can refer you to physicians in your area.

Appendix G provides an extensive, yet very incomplete, listing
of CFS, fibromyalgia, and related groups around the country.
Also check your local telephone directory as well as area health
food stores and libraries for additional groups. Another resource is your pharmacist, who is probably extremely familiar
with a good number of local physicians and their specialties.

One of the benefits of using a recommended physician, or a
wholistic physician, is that he or she is more likely to be familiar
with the approaches I discuss in this book. This will, of course,
make things much easier for you. A knowledgeable physician, or
a willing physician who has read this book, will have an organized
approach to treating your illness. Such a physician may also be

comfortable doing the counseling that is important for anyone with a disabling condition.

Your Insurance Also Plays a Role

The type of health insurance that you have may also play a role in your selection of a physician. Although some health maintenance organizations (HMOs) are excellent and very interested in their patients' well-being, some seem to be interested only in making money. When the latter is the case, the HMO may readily approve of tests and treatments that are clear-cut and lifesaving but, unfortunately, may drag its feet on allowing new treatment approaches, claiming they are experimental. There are, indeed, few readily accepted tests for chronic fatigue syndrome and fibromyalgia. If, however, you have any of the symptoms listed in Table 8.1, you can push for, and are legally entitled to have, the appropriate tests, listed beside the symptoms. The main tests to push for are those listed as most important on page 108 in Appendix A. Although the tests listed as helpful on that same page offer valuable information, they are less likely to be useful in the hands of a disinterested physician. Except for the stool testing, which you may find worthwhile to have done at my lab (see page 48) or at the Great Smoky Mountain Lab (see Appendix I), all of the tests can be effectively done anywhere. Again, you should review the results with page 109 in front of you. Otherwise, your physician may dismiss as "within normal limits" levels that are abnormal and contribute to your CFS.

If your physician is *capitated*—that is, if he or she is paid a set monthly fee by the insurance carrier for every patient, whether every patient is seen or not—that physician may lose money on every test ordered. This creates a perverse incentive for the physician not to do anything—and to hope that sick people go away. If your insurance company pays physicians a *fee for service*—payment based on the care provided—you stand the best chance of getting the help you need.

You must be courteous yet firm in your desires. Most physicians are very compassionate and want to help their patients. You must not be hostile when you first ask your doctor to try my treatment approach. At the same time, though, you must stand up for your needs.

As medicine becomes more competitive, *groups* of patients might be able to interest physicians in their cases. CFIDS and fibromyalgia support groups in an area can discuss which physicians seem the most interested, competent, and caring. A physician who is fee for service or who has a family member or personal experience with CFS or fibromyalgia will most likely be much more interested, since capitated physicians and physicians connected with HMOs would be committing financial suicide by seeking out sick patients. Representatives of the patient group can then approach the selected physician, in person or by letter, to see if the physician would be willing to treat the group members using the desired treatment approach. Let the physician know how many patients in the group would be interested in seeing him or her.

If your insurance company does not give you a choice of physicians, and your physician has no interest in running the tests that you need, you may have to file an appeal with the insurance company and with the state insurance commissioner. Unfortunately, you may also need to find legal assistance. Again, remember that you are not requesting the tests for *diagnosis* of CFS or fibromyalgia. The tests are in response to your symptoms (see Table 8.1). If your physician still refuses to do the testing, make sure that he or she has recorded all your symptoms in your chart, has described how incapacitating they are, and has noted the refusal to order the tests despite your strong requests. Then ask for copies of the progress notes in your chart that document these points. With these notes in hand, you may be able to receive reimbursement from your insurance company (on appeal) if you must pay to have the tests done by a *nonparticipating* physician. Getting into a hostile fight with a close-minded physician is not worth your while. Simply take the necessary steps to protect your rights.

Fighting your physician or insurance company is not a good use of your precious energy. In the long run, you will do better grouping together with other CFIDS patients to find physicians who will work with you. Remember, CFS, fibromyalgia, and other chronic fatigue states are now treatable illnesses. You will do best using your energy to find a physician who wants to work with you to help you move beyond your disease.

Table 8.1. Tests for Symptoms

If you have any of these symptoms	You have the right to have these tests done
Fatigue, abdominal discomfort, confusion	Complete blood count (CBC) and erythrocyte sedimentation rate (ESR) and differential
Fatigue, abdominal discomfort, confusion, recurrent infections	Chemistry (for example, chemistry 16 or chemistry 25) and magnesium
Anemia *or* fatigue	Iron (Fe), total iron binding capacity (TIBC), *and* ferritin (all three iron studies are necessary)
Fatigue, constipation or diarrhea, achiness, confusion, cold intolerance, sweating, palpitations	Thyroid studies including free or total T_3, free T_4, *and* thyroid-stimulating hormone (TSH) (all three tests are necessary)
Anemia, confusion, poor memory, fatigue, or paresthesia (numbness or tingling in the fingers)	Vitamin B_{12}
Malabsorption (for example, bowel distention or gas) or anemia	Folate
Increased thirst or urination	$HgbA_1C$ (diabetes screen) or glycosylated hemoglobin
Chronic diarrhea or abdominal cramps, gas, bloating, or other gastrointestinal complaints	Stool for ova and parasites, with antigen testing for amoeba, giardia, *Cryptosporidium*, and *Clostridia difficile*
Chronic muscle aches or joint aches	Creatine phosphokinase (CPK), antinuclear antibody (ANA), latex fixation (rheumatoid factor)
Fatigue, recurrent infections	Human immunodeficiency virus (HIV)
Vaginitis, confusion, rash	Rapid plasma reagin (RPR) (syphilis test)
Fatigue, achiness, joint pains, confusion, or poor memory	Lyme disease (necessary only in certain regions)
Runny nose, recurrent respiratory infections, nasal congestion, rashes, wheezing	Allergy testing and immunoglobulin E (IgE)
Under- or overactive thyroid (often helpful in interpreting the significance of borderline results)	Thyroid antibodies
Irregular or absent periods or hot flashes (check for menopause)	Follicle-stimulating hormone (FSH), luteinizing hormone (LH)
Decreased libido (in male or female), decreased erections	Testosterone and free testosterone

If you have any of these symptoms	You have the right to have these tests done
Abnormal body-hair growth, fatigue, or infertility	Dehydroepiandrosterone-sulfate (DHEA-S)
Fatigue, hypotension, or recurrent infections	Cortrosyn stimulation test (for adrenal insufficiency)
Fatigue with snoring, overweight, or periods of apnea	Sleep study
Chronic sinusitis	Sinus computed tomography (CT) scan

Important Points

- If your physician is not willing to treat you for CFS, find one who is by asking your friends and family for recommendations. Other good resources are local support groups, health food stores, libraries, and pharmacists.

- Check your health insurance regarding your rights in selecting a physician, having testing done, and getting treatment.

- Consider banding together with other CFIDS patients to interest a physician.

Conclusion

Old mindsets are often difficult to change. It took many years for chronic fatigue syndrome and fibromyalgia to be recognized as real and physical processes. As time goes on and more physicians become aware of these illnesses, patients will no longer have to accept being labeled as crazy because of the medical profession's ignorance.

We are now entering the next stage.

Chronic fatigue syndrome and fibromyalgia are now treatable. This simple fact needs to be demonstrated and reported over and over again to become accepted by physicians. The controlled study that I recently began on my treatment approach should help. Over time, more physicians will learn how to treat chronic fatigue and how to encourage and support their fatigue patients. Others, sadly, will continue to keep their heads stuck in the sand. It is alright to ignore these doctors who ignore you. You will be better off spending your energy tending to and taking responsibility for your physical and emotional needs so that you can attain and then maintain optimum health.

Because your illness may have been treated as being "all in your head" for so long, do not fall into the trap of ignoring your emotional and psychological needs. Many CFS patients were overachievers in an effort to compensate for childhood low self-esteem. *Love yourself* for having had that low self-esteem, *love yourself* for having been an overachiever, then let go of both these experiences. Take the "shoulds" placed on you by your family and society—you *should* be a mother, you *should* be a lawyer, you *should* do this, you *should* be that—and drop them. Love yourself for having had them, then love yourself for letting go of them. Although CFS is devastating, even this dark cloud has a silver lining. It has taught you what you do not have to do and has given you space to explore who you truly are. You have earned the right.

As you start feeling better, *slowly* add activities to your life that make you feel good. If you add something that makes you feel poorly, stop doing it. Joseph Campbell, a world-renowned teacher of the mythology of and paths for personal growth in many diverse cultures, was asked how people can stay true to themselves. Put succinctly, his advice was to "follow your bliss." Perhaps a "should" led you to become an accountant, doctor, or lawyer, but your bliss truly lies in being an artist, poet, or dancer. Perhaps the opposite is true. If you do what makes you feel happy and excited, you will get yourself on the right track. Whatever you do, however, *do not try to make up for lost time*. The few lingering symptoms of your illness will effectively let you know when you are pushing too hard. Recognize that your illness may have been a valuable teacher.

As your chronic fatigue resolves and you begin to feel well again, let your friends and former physicians (most CFS patients see quite a few!) know. Because no single expensive drug exists for the treatment of CFS, millions of pharmaceutical dollars are not spent on publicity. As you get well, that part—letting other fatigue patients know that an end to the tunnel does exist—is up to you.

Appendix A

For Physicians

The medical management of chronic fatigue syndrome (CFS) and fibromyalgia is, in many ways, fairly straightforward. Because the lab testing needs to be done and interpreted somewhat differently than for other conditions, I recommend reading this entire book. If time does not allow this, I recommend reading my study on CFS treatment, published in the Winter 1995 issue of the *Journal of Musculoskeletal Pain* (see Appendix B: Effective Treatment of Severe Chronic Fatigue: A Report of a Series of 64 Patients). This will help you understand the rationale behind my approach and will give you a good overview of what occurs in CFS.

The major physical components of CFS and fibromyalgia are the following:

- *Hypothalamic dysfunction.* Hypothalamic dysfunction, or autoimmune injury, often causes adrenal and thyroid underactivity. Current evidence suggests that vasopressin suppression is also common. Follicle-stimulating hormone (FSH) and luteinizing hormone (LH) may also be low.[1-6]

- *Immune dysfunction.* Immune dysfunction has been documented in CFS.[1] In fact, CFS is now called chronic fatigue and *immune dysfunction* syndrome (CFIDS). The immune dysfunction may result in *recurrent infections*, often with normally nonpathogenic organisms such as *Candida albicans* or bowel parasites.[7,8]

- *Nutritional inadequacies.* Nutritional deficiencies—especially of the B-complex vitamins, magnesium, or iron—may be aggravated by malabsorption or increased utilization.[9-14]

- *Fibromyalgia.* Fibromyalgia is a sleep disorder associated with multiple tender points. Hypothalamic dysfunction, immune dysfunction, and nutritional inadequacies can all cause or perpetuate myofascial pain syndromes and fibromyalgia.[9] Fibromyalgia may also *cause* hypothalamic and immune dysfunction.[2]

These four underlying problems need to be treated simultaneously, otherwise a vicious cycle can be kicked into action in which each problem can trigger the others. I call this cycle the "fatigue cycle." (See Figure A.1.)

An Approach to Chronic Fatigue Syndrome

In the following sections, I will present my approach to what I call severe chronic fatigue states. For summaries of the information, see pages 93, 108, 109, and 114.

PATIENT HISTORY

The symptoms and signs needed for the diagnosis of CFS are presented on page 7. These criteria, however, are more helpful as a research tool than as a clinical tool. In practice, the key questions are whether the patient has disabling fatigue, diffuse achiness that is worse with exercise, disordered sleep, brain fog (decreased memory and/or concentration), and perhaps increased thirst, all for more than six months. If these symptoms are persistent and the patient does not have other untreated organic problems—such as anemia, cancer, diabetes, lupus, polymyalgia rheumatica (PMR), or a chronic infection such as sinusitis or Lyme disease—the approach presented here will likely help. CFS and fibromyalgia are not "all or nothing" problems. Like arthritis and many other illnesses, they occur in varying degrees of severity. (See Appendix E: Fibromyalgia Information Questionnaire.)

PHYSICAL EXAMINATION

The same as patients with other disabling diseases, CFS patients must be given thorough physical examinations. Look for palpable nodes in the neck and axillae. These nodes should be smaller

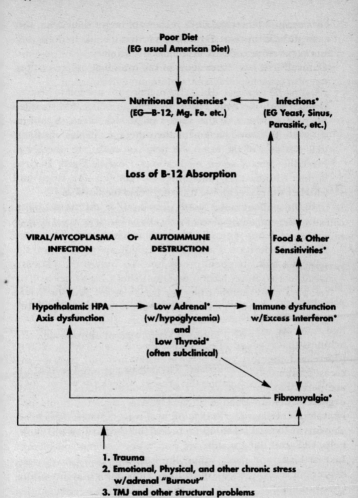

Figure A.1. The fatigue cycle.

than 2 centimeters (cm), since if they are larger than 2 cm, they are an indication that some other process is likely occurring. Pharyngeal, nonexudative erythema is common.

Clinically, several other areas of the examination are critical.

- *Check for fibromyalgia.* Time and practice are needed to become familiar with the tender point examination. The criteria listed on page 95 describe the tender points for which to look to diagnose fibromyalgia. Fortunately, the main clinical decisions that this part of the exam will help you make are whether to prescribe one of seven medications—Flexeril, Elavil, Desyrel, Soma, Klonopin, Dramamine, or Ambien—for sleep and whether to try an empiric trial of thyroid medication.

  If the patient notes poor sleep and/or diffuse achiness, prescribe one of the above medications for sleep regardless of the exam result. You should also consider a trial of low-dose thyroid medication if achiness or fatigue are present or if the patient's basal temperature is low. To obtain the patient's basal temperature, have the patient check his or her axillary temperature every morning for five to seven days for five to ten minutes before getting out of bed. A normal temperature is over 97.4°F.

  For a listing of additional symptoms of fibromyalgia for which to look, see Appendix E.

- *Check for thyroid tenderness.* Thyroiditis, or even borderline thyromegaly, is occasionally present. Check for a slow ankle deep tendon reflex relaxation phase.

- *Look for skin, nail, or vaginal signs of yeast or fungal infection.* A yeast or fungal infection increases the index of suspicion for bowel yeast overgrowth.

- *Check for nasal or sinus congestion, polyps, or septal deviation.* If a nasal or sinus problem is present, consider a trial of sinusitis or nasal-blockage treatment.[15] A treatment trial recommended by Dr. Alexander C. Chester III, a physician practicing in Washington, D.C., who is a strong advocate of nasal congestion and sinusitis as causes of chronic fatigue, is outlined on page 67. I also recommend trying the measures to combat a respiratory infection that are presented on page 47.

American College of Rheumatology 1990 Criteria for the Classification of Fibromyalgia*

HISTORY OF WIDESPREAD PAIN

Definition: Pain is considered widespread when all of the following are present:

- Pain in the left side of the body
- Pain in the right side of the body
- Pain above the waist
- Pain below the waist
- Axial skeletal pain (cervical spine or anterior chest or thoracic spine or low back)

In this definition, shoulder and buttock pain is considered pain for each involved side. "Low back" pain is considered lower segment pain.

PAIN IN 11 OF 18 TENDER POINT SITES ON DIGITAL PALPATION†

Definition: Pain on digital palpation, must be present in at least 11 of the following 18 tender point sites.

- Occiput: Bilateral, at the suboccipital muscle insertions
- Low cervical: Bilateral, at the anterior aspects of the intertransverse spaces at C5–C7
- Trapezius: Bilateral, at the midpoint of the upper border
- Supraspinatus: Bilateral, at origins, above the scapular spine near the medial border
- Second rib: Bilateral, at the second costochondral junctions, just lateral to the junctions on upper surfaces
- Lateral epicondyle: Bilateral, 2 cm distal to the epicondyles

---

- Gluteal: Bilateral, in upper outer quadrants of buttocks in anterior fold of muscle
- Greater trochanter: Bilateral, posterior to the trochanteric prominence
- Knees: Bilateral, at the medial fat pad proximal to the joint line

*For classification purposes, patients are said to have fibromyalgia if both criteria are satisfied. Widespread pain must have been present for at least 3 months. The presence of a second clinical disorder does not exclude the diagnosis of fibromyalgia.

†Digital palpation should be performed with an approximate force of 4 kg. For tender point to be considered positive, the subject must state that the palpation was "painful," a reply of "tender" is not to be considered painful.

From F. Wolfe, et al , "The American College of Rheumatology 1990 Criteria for the Classification of Fibromyalgia· Report of the Multicenter Criteria Committee," *Arthritis and Rheumatology* 33 (1990)· 160–172. Used with permission.

- *Look for a coated tongue.* A coated tongue, as opposed to each taste bud being an individual white "dot," suggests a B-vitamin deficiency, which usually resolves after taking a multivitamin high in the B vitamins for three to six months. Inflammation of individual taste buds that comes and goes is part of the same process. Tongue fissuring is suggestive of severe, long-standing B-vitamin deficiency and takes four to five years to resolve, although the patient may feel better quickly. A smooth tongue suggests deficiency of the B vitamins or iron.

- *Check for mitral valve prolapse.* Magnesium treatment is important for all CFS patients, but it is especially important for patients with mitral valve prolapse.

Some researchers recommend also looking for a crimson crest on the soft palate. However, a crimson crest is common even in healthy patients, so I do not find it to be a useful sign.

LAB TESTING

Many approaches exist to lab testing in CFS. Some physicians recommend very little testing, preferring instead to just reassure patients that they are not dying and send them home as untreatable. However, not checking for treatable processes guarantees continued disability.

I recommend a fair amount of testing, but I limit it to tests that can lead to helping the patient recover. The tests that I find most important, as well as the tests that I find helpful, are listed on page 108. As noted previously, tests that come back as normal may still indicate a need for treatment. The interpretation of some tests is self-evident. However, the correct interpretation of others is critical to your patient's improvement. (See page 109 for a guide to interpreting tests in CFS.)

Among available tests, I have found the following to be useful:

- *Free or total T₃, free T₄, and thyroid-stimulating hormone (TSH).* If the T_3 or T_4 test results are even just on the low side of normal, I sometimes consider an empiric trial of Synthroid, 25 to 50 micrograms (mcg) every morning (q.a.m.), or Armour Thyroid, .25 to 1 grain q.a.m. I am more likely to try an empiric trial of thyroid-hormone therapy if one or more of the following is true:

  - the patient has fibromyalgia.

  - the patient's morning basal axillary temperature is generally less than 97.4°F.

  - the patient has symptoms and signs suggestive of hypothyroidism.

  - the patient's TSH test result is less than .95 or greater than 3.0.

  Physicians are trained to interpret a low-normal TSH—that is, .5 to .95—as a confirmation of euthyroidism. The rules, however, are different with CFS. In this setting, hypothalamic hypothyroidism is common and the patient's TSH can be low, normal, or high.[16] This is why I recommend an empiric therapeutic trial of thyroid-hormone treatment if the TSH and T_4 are both low normal. Also, if subclinical hypothyroidism is missed, the patient's fibromyalgia simply will not resolve.

  In addition, I would add the following:

  - If the patient does not respond to Synthroid, switch to

Armour Thyroid, and vice versa. For every 50 mcg of Synthroid, have the patient take .5 grain of Armour Thyroid. If the free or total T_3 result is low or low normal, try Armour Thyroid, which has both T_3 and T_4, instead of Synthroid, which has only T_4.

- Adjust the thyroid dose according to how the patient feels and also to get a basal temperature greater than 98°F. This is as long as the T_3 or T_4 tests do not show hyperthyroidism.

- Make sure that the patient does not take any iron supplements within six hours of the morning thyroid dose or the thyroid hormone will not be absorbed.[17] Have the patient take the iron at night and away from any hormone treatments.

- Thyroid supplementation can increase a patient's cortisol metabolism and unmask a mild adrenal insufficiency. If the patient feels worse on low-dose thyroid replacement, the patient may have adrenal (or thiamine) insufficiency.

Remember that every patient is an individual and will respond differently to medications.

- *Thyroid antibodies (antimicrosomal and antithyroglobulan antibodies).* Autoimmune and other forms of thyroiditis sometimes trigger fatigue. Positive antibodies and low-normal T_3 or T_4 results, especially with fibromyalgia, strongly suggest that a therapeutic trial of thyroid-hormone treatment may help.

- *Magnesium level.* Serum magnesium does not drop until the body's muscle stores are at least one-third depleted.[18,19] This can perhaps be considered as equivalent to 2.8 being the lower limit of normal on potassium testing. I treat all fatigue patients with magnesium malate, chloride, or lactate. Two good products are Slow-Mag and Mag-Tab SR, which are both available over-the-counter (OTC) at pharmacies. I now prefer using magnesium with malic acid, also known as magnesium malate, since it is more effective than magnesium chloride or lactate.[20] The recommended dosage for all three is two tablets three times a day (t.i.d.) for eight months, then two tablets once a day (q.d.). Magnesium malate is available by mail order as

Fibrocare or Super Malic (see Appendix I: Mail Order Sources). If the patient gets diarrhea, decrease the dose.

- *Erythrocyte sedimentation rate (ESR).* This level is usually low, for example, less than 6 with fibromyalgia and CFS. PMR mimics fibromyalgia but will show a high ESR, as will lupus and other inflammatory diseases.

- *Complete blood count (CBC) with differential.* If the mean cell volume (MCV) is greater than 93 in the absence of alcohol abuse, I would more strongly consider thyroid and/or B_{12} treatment. If the eosinophil count is elevated, I would look more closely for asthma, allergies, or bowel parasites, although parasites are commonly seen even with a normal eosinophil count.

- *Iron (Fe), total iron binding capacity (TIBC), ferritin.* I have diagnosed several cases of biopsy-proven hemochromatosis whose only symptom was fatigue. Elevated ferritin with a percent saturation greater than 50 percent would be an indication to explore this further. If the ferritin is *less than* 40 nanograms per milliliter (ng/ml) or the percent saturation is *less than* 22 percent, prescribe Chromagen (a prescription iron), Ferrous-Sequels, or Vitron C, one tablet once a day (q.d.) or twice a day (b.i.d.) for four to six months. Make sure to instruct the patient not to take this medication within four to six hours of any thyroid hormone. Although a ferritin level greater than 9 ng/ml prevents anemia, it may not be adequate for other body functions.[21,22]

- *Vitamin B_{12} level.* Although technically normal if greater than 208 picograms per milliliter (pg/ml), studies show that B_{12} deficiency can cause severe neuropsychiatric changes even at much higher levels.[23] Although current normal levels prevent anemia, they do not prevent neurologic injury. Recent Framingham data suggest that B_{12} deficiency, determined by metabolic testing, can exist even with levels greater than 540 pg/ml.[24] If the patient's B_{12} level is *less than* 540 pg/ml, I recommend vitamin B_{12} injections, 1 milligram (mg) intramuscularly (IM) once a week for a total of eight to ten injections. Although these injections are controversial, they are also safe, inexpensive, and often very helpful. Many patients need only about eight B_{12} shots before seeing improvement. If improvement occurs but fades when the shots are stopped, resume the shots weekly until the patient feels better and then give one shot every one to five weeks as needed. Trying an empiric trial of B_{12} injections, regardless of the B_{12} level, is reasonable.[25]

● *Stool for ova and parasites (O&P), giardia, Clostridia difficile, Cryptosporidium, amoebic antibodies, white blood cells (WBC), and quantitative yeast.* These tests are very helpful. I frequently find patients whose disabling fatigue *dramatically* resolves after they are treated for bowel parasites. Although many CFS patients have spastic colon–like symptoms, many patients with bowel parasites have no bowel symptoms. Because of their immune dysfunction, CFS patients benefit from treating parasites that are even considered nonpathogenic. *Cryptosporidium* and other parasites can be treated with the herb *Artemisia annua*, 1 gram (gm) t.i.d. for twenty days. Dr. Leo Galland, a parasite specialist, recommends tricyclin, two tablets t.i.d. for six to eight weeks. Tricyclin is a Chinese herbal remedy that is available by mail order (see Appendix I). Approximately one in eight fatigue patients tests positive for stool parasites.

Although no good test has as yet been developed for stool fungal overgrowth, making this a controversial area, I find that quantifying stool yeast levels on O&P is very helpful.

Most labs do not find parasites in the stool even if parasites are present.[26] Patients need to take one and a half ounces of Fleets Phospho-Soda laxative and provide three loose stool samples. You must have your O&Ps tested in a lab that *specializes* in parasitology. If such a lab is not available in your area, you can have the stool tests done by mail in my lab. To order a test kit containing the necessary forms, instructions, and specimen containers, contact me at the address listed in Appendix I. When the testing is completed, my lab will send a copy of the results and treatment recommendations to both you and your patient. Great Smoky Mountain Lab (see Appendix I) also does a very good job with stool testing.

● *Serum amoeba antibodies.* Cysts are passed intermittently and O&Ps may miss amoebic infections. Testing for serum amoeba antibodies is helpful as a backup. If amoebic infection is suspected based on the testing, consider Flagyl, 750 mg by mouth (p.o.) t.i.d. for ten days, followed by Yodoxin, 650 mg t.i.d. for twenty more days. If the patient cannot tolerate the Flagyl, reduce the dose.

- *Creatine phosphokinase (CPK).* This screens for dermatomyositis, polymyositis, and other muscle disorders.

- *Cortrosyn stimulation test.* This test, which checks adrenal function, is a critical test in CFS. It can be done in your office or at a lab. It is important that the cortisol baseline be drawn between 7:30 and 8:30 A.M. After checking the baseline cortisol, give the patient 25 international units (IU) of adrenocorticotropic hormone (ACTH), or cortrosyn, IM and check cortisol levels at thirty minutes and one hour. I consider a trial of Cortef treatment to be worthwhile if:

  - The cortisol level at baseline is less than 12 micrograms per deciliter (mcg/dl), *or*

  - The cortisol level does not increase by at least 7 mcg/dl at thirty minutes and 11 mcg/dl at one hour, *or*

  - The cortisol level does not double from the baseline and is under 35 to 40 mcg/dl.

No consensus exists on the test's interpretation. Some experts consider the test positive if any of the above criteria are met. Others consider as normal any test in which either the cortisol baseline is over 6 mcg/dl or the level goes over 20 mcg/dl.

Dr. William Jeffries, a retired professor of endocrinology at Case-Western Reserve Medical School, has been researching cortisol treatment for chronic fatigue states for many decades. He recommends an empiric trial of Cortef, approximately 5 to 7.5 mg three times a day (t.i.d.) to four times a day (q.i.d.), in all cases of severe unexplained fatigue.[27,28] This is because:

- Strict interpretation of the cortrosyn stimulation test misses many cases of disabling, suboptimal adrenal function.

- The low doses of Cortef recommended are fairly safe.[29]

- CFS patients often experience dramatic improvement with low-dose Cortef.[28]
- Hypothalamic-pituitary-adrenal axis dysfunction has been demonstrated in chronic fatigue patients.[1-6]

My treatment guidelines are that if the baseline cortisol is less than 12 mcg/dl, treat with 5 mg Cortef t.i.d. with meals. If the baseline cortisol is greater than 11 mcg/dl but does not increase by 7 mcg/dl at thirty minutes *and* 11 mcg/dl at one hour, or does not double by one hour and remains at less than 40 mcg/dl, treat with 5 mg Cortef in the morning and 2.5 mg at lunchtime and increase to 5 mg p.o. t.i.d. as needed.

After keeping the patient on the initial dose for two to four weeks, adjust the dose up to a maximum of 30 mg daily or, if no benefit has been evident, taper it off. Give most of the Cortef in the morning and at lunchtime. I often tell my patients to take the last dose, 2.5 to 5 mg, no later than 4 P.M. Otherwise, the Cortef may keep the patient up at night.

After six to twelve months, taper the Cortef off over a period of one to two months and perhaps repeat the cortrosyn test. If the other physiologic stresses, such as infections or fibromyalgia, have been eliminated, the patient's adrenal function may be adequate or normalized.

Improvement is often dramatic and is usually seen within two weeks. The Cortef should be doubled during periods of acute stress and raised even higher during periods of severe stress such as surgery. Consider also giving the patient 1,000 mg of calcium and 400 IU of vitamin D daily with the Cortef.

Being a center for CFS research, my office has been invited by a research team from the National Institutes of Health (NIH) to contribute patients to a currently ongoing controlled study using Cortef, 37.5 mg daily, in all patients with CFS. This NIH group has done excellent work in CFS. However, I am concerned that by not treating the other factors causing the chronic fatigue, these researchers may miss many of Cortef's treatment benefits.

- *Glycosylated hemoglobin (HgbA₁C).* Although this diabetes screen is not very specific, it is helpful in testing for hypoglycemia. Hypoglycemia is most often caused by inadequate adrenal function.[28] If the results are less than 5.4, a trial of low-dose Cortef may help even if the cortrosyn test is borderline. This test also, of course, screens for diabetes.

- *Dehydroepiandrosterone-sulfate (DHEA-S) level.* DHEA is a major adrenal hormone. Low levels of it are associated with shorter life spans.[30] If the DHEA-S level is under 150 mcg/dl in a female or 350 mcg/dl in a male, I recommend a therapeutic trial of DHEA treatment. (For normal DHEA-S ranges, based on patients' sex and age, see Table A.1.) CFS patients often have improved energy when treated with DHEA, 5 to 60 mg q.d.[31] Adjust the dose to keep the DHEA-S level at no lower than 150 mcg/dl. Recheck the DHEA-S level every two to four months as a matter of course and six weeks after any dosing change.

  Interestingly, as patients improve, their bodies begin to make DHEA on their own and the DHEA-S level can shoot up. If the level goes too high, the patient can get acne or darkening of the facial hair. Because of this, it is reasonable to check the DHEA-S level every two months in a female or every three to four months in a male. Although the body's DHEA-S level is fairly stable throughout the day, which is why I check the DHEA-sulfate level as opposed to the more variable DHEA level, the DHEA-S level does show marked peaks and troughs when DHEA is taken by mouth. I strongly recommend either prescribing time-release DHEA or using b.i.d.–t.i.d. dosing. When the DHEA-S level rises over 200 mcg/dl in a female or 450 mcg/dl in a male, start to taper the dose. It takes four to six weeks to reach a new steady-state dose after a dosing change.

  DHEA is available by mail order (see Appendix I).

- *Automated chemistry profile (chem 19) and urinalysis (UA) with microscopic exam.* These tests screen for liver, kidney, and other metabolic problems.

- *Antinuclear antibody (ANA) and latex fixation.* These tests screen for lupus, rheumatoid arthritis, and other connective tissue diseases that can cause secondary fibromyalgia.

- *Lyme titer, human immunodeficiency virus (HIV), rapid plasma reagin (RPR).* Lyme disease, HIV, and syphilis can cause chronic fatigue and fibromyalgia. False positive Lyme titers

Table A.1. Normal DHEA-S Levels (mcg/dl)

	Age Group	Fifth Percentile	Fiftieth Percentile	Ninety-Fifth Percentile
Females	10–19	–	140	–
	20–29	65	185	380
	30–39	45	150	270
	40–49	32	120	240
	50–59	26	85	200
	60–69	13	50	130
	70–79	17	40	90
	80–89	–	26	–
	Postmenopausal	10	55	190
Males	10–19	–	215	–
	20–29	280	420	640
	30–39	120	300	520
	40–49	95	250	530
	50–59	70	160	310
	60–69	42	130	290
	70–79	28	80	175
	80–89	–	36	–

Many experts recommend keeping the DHEA-S level at the fiftieth percentile for a twenty-nine-year-old. If hirsutism occurs in females or acne in males or females, decrease the dose.

are common and must be confirmed by other testing and by clinical setting.

- *FSH and LH.* Check if menopause is a consideration. Some women display early menopause even with regular periods. In these women, night sweats can interfere with sleep and cause fatigue. Treatment with Premarin or the natural estrogen triestrogen has at times resulted in dramatic improvement. Triestrogen is available by mail order (see Appendix I). When prescribing it, keep in mind that 2.5 mg is equivalent to .625 mg of Premarin.
- *Immunoglobulin E (IgE) and allergy testing.* Run these tests if you suspect allergies.
- *Tuberculosis skin test.*
- *Sinus computed tomography (CT) scan.* Consider this test if chronic sinusitis is present and if it persists despite treatment.

- *Sleep testing.* Run this test if you suspect sleep apnea or restless leg syndrome. Sleep apnea is more likely if the patient is overweight or snores.

- *Yeast questionnaire.* No definitive test as yet exists to differentiate normal yeast growth from overgrowth. Therefore, I have my patients fill out the yeast questionnaire that was devised by Dr. William G. Crook and that is presented in Appendix D. Suspect yeast overgrowth if the patient either gets a high score on the questionnaire or shows yeast overgrowth on the stool microscopic exam. Often dramatically helpful is an empiric trial of nystatin, two 500,000-IU tablets p.o. q.i.d. (start slowly) for five months, with Diflucan or Sporanox, 100 mg once a day for one week, followed by 200 mg each morning for five weeks. The patient's symptoms, especially fibromyalgia pain, may flare initially as the yeast die off. Therefore, begin with one 500,000-IU tablet nystatin once a day and increase by one tablet every one to three days, as tolerated, up to two tablets q.i.d. Some physicians feel that nystatin is more effective in powder form than in tablets. After four weeks on the nystatin, add the Diflucan or Sporanox as described above. The other major side effect of both Diflucan and Sporanox is the price—a six-week course can cost more than $500. If symptoms *recur* after the first six weeks on Diflucan or Sporanox, I recommend returning to 200 mg per day for another six weeks. If no benefit is derived from the first course, I do not recommend repeating it. Have your patient stay on the nystatin for a total of five to eight months.

    Sporanox must be taken with food and stomach acid to be properly absorbed. Acid blockers such as Zantac and Maalox will prevent its absorption. Diflucan does not require stomach acid for proper absorption. *Do not use Seldane, Hismanal, or Propulcid with Diflucan or Sporinox, as the combination can cause fatal arrhythmias.* Claritin can be used. Sweets must also be avoided, since they seem to stimulate yeast growth. One cup of yogurt with live and active yogurt cultures eaten daily is helpful. Refrigerated acidophilus bacteria, 4 billion IU per day, also can help to restore normal bowel flora.

- *Free testosterone level.* Testosterone levels are often low in CFS patients and should be checked. Make sure that your lab gives you normal ranges based on your patients' ages. If the levels are low, 200 mg of testosterone IM every two weeks can help male patients dramatically, while .25 mg of methyltestosterone p.o. q.d. to t.i.d. can do the same for female patients.

- *Elimination diet.* If a patient's symptoms persist despite treatment, food allergies may be the problem.

Many excellent physicians also check viral and immune titers such as interferon and interleukin titers. At this time, the results of these tests would not affect my treatment or diagnosis. Therefore, I do not run the tests.

In the future, testing for insulin stimulated growth hormone levels may help in nonresponders.

GENERAL TREATMENT

The general regimen that I recommend in addition to the specific treatments outlined under Lab Testing includes the following:

- TwinLab Daily One Caps, available OTC, or Berocca Plus vitamins, available by prescription, one daily. Both these multivitamins make the urine turn bright yellow. Whichever one you use, direct the patient to take it with food because it may cause nausea. If you choose the Berocca Plus vitamins, prescribe the generic, since it costs $15 for one hundred tablets versus $50 for one hundred of the brand name.

- Magnesium chloride (Slow-Mag) or magnesium lactate (Mag-Tab SR), available OTC, or magnesium malate (Fibrocare), available by mail order (see Appendix I), two tablets t.i.d.

- No sweets for six months. This includes nondiet soft drinks.

- No caffeine or alcohol for six months.

- Therapeutic counseling to uncover any life conflicts. I recommend the Jungian approach.

- Exercise, slowly at first. I tell my patients to begin with walking and to advance as they are able. If the patient feels worse the next day, I tell the patient to go easier at the next exercise session.

- No antibiotics if possible. Erythromycin and Macrodantin seem to cause the least yeast overgrowth.

- Sleep eight hours per night.

In addition to the above recommendations, I encourage my patients not to try to make up for lost time when they begin to feel better. They may not be able to return to work for an extended period no matter how well they feel.

Additional Treatment Approaches

Some of the following are treatments that I use and recommend in addition to the specific and general treatments thus far discussed. Some are treatments used by other physicians and are also highly recommended. Remember, for a patient's CFS to resolve, all the patient's problems must be treated simultaneously.

- *Treat the fibromyalgia.* Treating the problems that we have already discussed is critical and often results in dramatic improvement in a patient's fibromyalgia. Also very helpful is *nonaddictive* medication to restore deep sleep. Fibromyalgia patients tend to be sensitive to medications. Therefore, start with a very low dose. The next-day sedation that most patients experience often resolves in two to three weeks. If it does not, have the patient take the medication earlier in the evening— for example, at around 7:00—so that it wears off earlier the next day.

    I do *not* recommend addictive sleeping pills. Addictive sleep remedies, except Klonopin, actually decrease the time that is spent in deep sleep and can worsen fibromyalgia.

    The medications that I do recommend include the following:

- *Elavil (amitriptyline), 10 mg.* Use one-half to five tablets at bedtime (q.h.s.). This medication is one of my first choices for most fibromyalgia patients.

- *Ambien (zolpidem), 5 to 10 mg.* Use 5 to 20 mg q.h.s. This medication is a newer agent with fewer side effects than the other medications. It is very helpful for most patients and is, along with Elavil, my first choice in medication.

Recommended Lab Tests

Most Important	Helpful

The following tests are the most important to order:

- Free or total T_3, free T_4, TSH
- Chem 19
- CBC with differential
- ESR
- Magnesium level
- Fe, TIBC, ferritin
- UA with micro
- Vitamin B_{12} level
- Stool for O&P, giardia, *Cryptosporidium*, *Clostridia difficile*, WBC, and quantitative yeast (see page 100)
- CPK
- Cortrosyn stimulation test
- Yeast questionnaire (see Appendix D)
- DHEA-S level
- IgE
- Stool and/or serum amoeba antibodies
- Free testosterone level (in males and females)

The following tests should be ordered according to the patient's needs:

- HIV
- ANA
- Thyroid antibodies (especially for patients with fibromyalgia)
- Lyme titer (if Lyme disease is common in your area)
- RPR
- Latex fixation
- $HgbA_1C$
- FSH and LH
- Allergy testing
- Sleep testing (if the patient is male or overweight, or if sleep apnea or restless leg syndrome is suspected)
- Sinus CT scan (if sinusitis persists despite treatment)
- PPD
- Elimination diet and/or blood tests for food sensitivities
- Folic acid level

For more information on these tests, see pages 96 to 106.

Selected Test Interpretations

The following tests need to be interpreted differently in CFIDS and fibromyalgia due to hypothalamic and immune dysfunction:

- *Thyroid testing.* Recheck free or total T_3 and free T_4 six weeks after changing medication.

  - *Free or total T_3.* If low normal, consider a trial of Armour Thyroid, .25 to 1 grain q.a.m.
  - *Free T_4.* If low normal, consider a trial of Synthroid, 25 mcg, one to three tablets q.a.m. If this treatment makes the patient feel worse, it may indicate adrenal insufficiency or euthyroidism, or thiamine deficiency (add 200 mg supplemental thiamine q.d.). If the treatment effects no change, consider changing to Armour Thyroid.
  - *TSH.* If greater than 3.0 or less than .9 (with a low normal T_3 or T_4), consider treatment as described above.
  - *Thyroid antibodies.* If positive, consider a trial of Synthroid, 25 to 75 mg q.a.m. (unless T_4 is high or high normal, in which case hyperthyroidism may be contributing to the fatigue), or Armour Thyroid, .25 to .75 grain q.a.m.

- *Cortrosyn stimulation test.* If the baseline cortisol is *less than* 12 mcg/dl or if the cortisol level does not double at one hour and is less than 35 to 40 mcg/dl, consider a trial of Cortef, 5 mg t.i.d. with meals. The Cortef can be adjusted up to as much as 30 mg per day and down to as little as 2.5 mg per day. Review the controversial nature of this treatment with the patient. If the patient is not diabetic or hypertensive, the main demonstrated risk at this dose is gastritis. Add calcium with vitamin D if the patient takes more than 15 mg of Cortef per day. Patients can often be weaned down or off the Cortef after three to nine months of feeling well. Taper by a half-tablet (2.5 mg) every one to two weeks.

- *Magnesium level.* I treat all fatigue patients with magnesium chloride or lactate, 67 mg, or, preferably, magnesium plus malic acid, two tablets t.i.d. for eight months and then two tablets q.d. If the magnesium level is *less than* 1.7, the magnesium stores may be low. Use less magnesium if diarrhea occurs or if the creatinine is elevated.

- *Vitamin B_{12} level.* I recommend a trial of B_{12}, 1 mg IM weekly for eight to ten weeks if the B_{12} level is less than 540 pg/ml or if the patient is not responding to other treatments. If the patient improves with this treatment but the effect wears off when the treatment is discontinued, continue 1 mg IM every one to four weeks as needed.

- *Stool tests.* I treat *all* parasites. If yeast overgrowth (1-plus or greater) is present *or* if the yeast questionnaire (see Appendix D) is positive, I treat with nystatin and either Sporanox or Diflucan.

- *Iron studies.* If the percent saturation is less than 22 percent *or* the ferritin level is less than 40 ng/ml, treat with iron. I recommend Chromagen or Ferrous-Sequels, one tablet b.i.d. Both of these formulas are less constipating than others. If not tolerated, an herbal iron formula, available at health food stores, may be helpful. *Make sure that the patient does not take the iron within four hours of thyroid medication or the thyroid medication will not be absorbed.*

- *DHEA-S level.* If low (less than 150 mcg/dl in females or 350 mcg/dl in males), consider a trial of DHEA, 5 to 50 mg p.o. q.d., to bring the DHEA-S level up. I like to keep patients in the fiftieth percentile for a twenty-nine-year-old. As patients improve, their natural DHEA often kicks back in and the supplement can cause high DHEA-S levels. This can result in acne or facial-hair darkening. I recommend checking DHEA-S levels approximately every two months in females and every three to four months in males. Adjust the DHEA treatment accordingly.

For more information on these tests, see pages 96 to 106.

- *Flexeril (cyclobenzaprine), 10 mg, and/or Soma, 350 mg.* Use one-half to one tablet q.h.s. Both medications are often very sedating. Use one of these first if myalgias are a major problem.

- *Desyrel (trazodone), 50 mg.* Use one-half to six tablets q.h.s. Use this medication first if anxiety is a major problem.

- *Health food store products.* If the patient does not tolerate medication very well, recommend 360 mg valerian root, 160 mg passionflower, and 160 mg lemon balm q.h.s. Also helpful is .3 mg melatonin q.h.s. Often, adding these to allow a lower dose of medication is also helpful.

For patients with disabling muscle aches, Klonopin can be very helpful. However, it has the potential to be somewhat addictive and very sedating, so I reserve it for patients with severe pain who do not respond to or tolerate any of the other medications. Begin with .25 mg q.h.s. and slowly adjust the dose upward as the next-day sedation diminishes.

Approximately 25 percent of fibromyalgia patients obtain about four hours relief from their achiness with sublingual nitroglycerin, .3 mg. Begin with one-half tablet or less. Headache is common initially but usually disappears after the first few tablets. Massage and *gentle* physical therapy or neuromuscular re-education, such as Trager therapy, can also be very helpful. In addition, a recent pilot study giving lidocaine, 240 mg intravenously (IV) over forty minutes (with the patient on a monitor) once a week for four weeks, resulted in marked improvement in eight of eleven patients.[32]

- *Treat any anxiety and/or depression.* CFIDS patients are often appropriately depressed or anxious because of their disabilities. Studies have shown that the depression is usually caused by the illness and that the illness is *not* caused by the depression.[5] This is true with any disabling illness. Fibromyalgia patients have low cerebrospinal-fluid serotonin levels. Antidepressants, which raise serotonin levels, have recently been proven to help fibromyalgia patients. Using Prozac, Zoloft, Serzone, Effexor, or Paxil can often improve a CFS patient's quality of life. Start with a low dose—for example, 10 mg of

Prozac—and slowly increase as needed. Desyrel, which often helps with anxiety, is not addictive.

- *Try coenzyme Q₁₀, 30 to 50 mg t.i.d.* Available OTC, coenzyme Q_{10} is sometimes helpful. However, effects may not be felt for four to five weeks.

- *Try evening primrose oil and fish oil.* Although I rarely use these, I have found that some patients benefit from two 500-mg capsules of evening primrose oil q.i.d. plus 1,000 mg of MaxEPA per day. Both are available OTC. It takes three months to see the full effect.

- *Treat any nasal congestion.* See page 67 for Dr. Chester's therapeutic treatment trial for nasal congestion and sinusitis.

- *If recurrent infections or severe fatigue persists,* consider an empiric trial of Gammar (gamma globulin), 4 to 5 cubic centimeters (cc) IM weekly for five weeks. After five weeks, decrease the dose.

- *If magnesium is less than 1.6,* consider magnesium sulfate, 2 gm IM four times a week for four weeks. To decrease soreness from the shot, add .1 cc of 2-percent lidocaine. Give 2 cc of a 50-percent solution (1 gm) in each buttock; do *not* use the 50-percent solution IV. Afterwards, have the patient wait in the office for thirty minutes to make sure dizziness does not occur. If dizziness does occur, have the patient lie down.

- *If the fibromyalgia persists,* add a daily dose of 1,000 to 1,500 mg of calcium with 400 to 1,000 IU of vitamin D. A recent study found high doses of 2,000 to 10,000 IU of vitamin D a day to help. However, it is critical to watch for hypercalcemia and vitamin D toxicity at these very high levels.

- *When all else fails,* Dr. Jay Goldstein has added many new tools. Dr. Goldstein is a Los Angeles physician who is a leading research expert on the role of neurotransmitters and central nervous system dysfunctions in CFS. In his book *Betrayal by the Brain* (see Appendix C: Recommended Reading), he discusses medications that often help CFS patients. Whether a medication will help an individual patient should be apparent within one hour of the first dose.[33] Because of this, empirically trying one dose of each medication, one at a time, each hour during symptomatic days is a reasonable approach. Stop when you find the medication that works. This testing is best done in your office under supervision, since CFS patients are often subject to medication side effects.

Among Dr. Goldstein's many recommendations are:

- *Cognex, 10 mg t.i.d. or q.i.d.* This is a centrally acting cholinesterase inhibitor. The patient's liver function will need to be tested on a weekly basis.

- *Nimodipine (Nimotop), 30 mg.* This is a calcium channel antagonist used for subarachnoid hemorrhages. Dr. Goldstein feels that it is the most beneficial medication that he currently uses.

- *Risperdal (risperidone), .25 to 1 mg b.i.d.* This is a serotonin (5-HT$_2$) receptor antagonist. At high doses, it is also a dopamine (D$_2$) receptor antagonist that is helpful in schizophrenia. For CFS, use very low doses.

- *Oxytocin, 10 IU p.o. q.d.* This is also a hypothalamic neurotransmitter[34] and is worth trying in a patient with pallor and cold extremities. Begin after the patient's DHEA has been normalized for three months. Dr. Jorge Fletchas, another CFS researcher, has also found oxytocin to be very useful. Effects can be seen in less than two weeks. Oxytocin can be purchased by mail order (see Appendix I).

- *Calan, 60 to 120 mg q.h.s.* This is in the same family as Nimotop but is much less expensive. If Nimotop works, try switching to Calan to help the patient save money.

For more of Dr. Goldstein's recommendations, see his book. Although Dr. Goldstein's multidimensional approach takes some time and practice to learn, I suspect that you will find it very helpful in treating your chronic fatigue patients. I would recommend, however, reading his book before using his protocol.

I would also recommend reading my study (see Appendix B) and the rest of this book as time goes on. For those physicians who would like more depth, I have listed some excellent books

Summary of Recommended Treatments

The following is a summary of the treatment regimen that I recommend for CFS:

- Treat nutritional deficiencies with TwinLab Daily One Caps or Berocca Plus multivitamins.
- Treat magnesium deficiency with magnesium chloride or lactate (Slow-Mag or Mag-Tab SR) or, preferably, magnesium with malic acid (Fibrocare).
- Do not allow any sweets, alcohol, or caffeine for three to six months, then limit them to moderate amounts. Expect withdrawal symptoms during the first week.
- Require at least eight hours of sleep a night.
- Recommend exercise, slowly at first, then more with improvement.
- Treat hypothyroidism with Synthroid or Armour Thyroid.
- Treat low or borderline adrenal function with Cortef and/or DHEA. If the patient is hypotensive, try Florinef. Monitor for hypokalemia.
- Consider treatment with estrogen in a female or testosterone in a male or female if levels are low.
- Treat any bowel infections.
- Treat any yeast overgrowth. Avoid antibiotics whenever possible.
- Treat any sinusitis or nasal congestion.
- Consider vitamin B_{12} injections once a week for at least eight to ten weeks.
- Treat fibromyalgia with low-dose Elavil, Desyrel, Flexeril, Soma, Ambien, or herbals to improve sleep.
- Consider treating anxiety with Desyrel at night.
- Consider treating depression or frustration with Paxil, Prozac, Serzone, Effexor, or Zoloft. These medications often help fibromyalgia even in the absence of depression.

- Treat unconscious life conflicts with counseling. I recommend Jungian, but there are many other excellent treatment approaches.
- Consider treating persistent fibromyalgia with sublingual nitroglycerin, Nimotop, calcium, and/or Klonopin.
- Consider treating persistent fatigue with coenzyme Q_{10}, evening primrose oil and fish oil, IM magnesium, and/or IM gamma globulin.
- Treat persistent CFS with Dr. Jay Goldstein's treatment protocol.

For full explanations of the individual items, see the appropriate sections within this appendix.

in a short list of recommended reading (see Appendix C). I think you will find it as exciting as I have to watch CFS and fibromyalgia patients turn vibrant!

Appendix B

Effective Treatment of Severe Chronic Fatigue: A Report of a Series of 64 Patients

Jacob Teitelbaum
Barbara Bird

ABSTRACT. Objectives: To determine the underlying causes of severe chronic fatigue states and the effect of concurrently treating the underlying etiologies.

Methods: Sixty-four patients with a median of three years of severe fatigue, which markedly limited their activity, were studied. These patients were characterized by a mix of symptoms including recurrent sore throats, swollen glands, increased thirst, sleeplessness, achiness, and poor memory and concentration without apparent cause. They presented in our office during 1991–1993 and were selected by consecutive sampling. The patients were assessed and treated for the processes noted below.

As fatigue is purely subjective, the patient determined if they showed worsening, no significant change, significant but incomplete improvement, or much improvement [i.e., fatigue no longer a problem].

Results: 46 patients had at least three or more contributing problems. Fibromyalgia was present in 44 patients. Overt or subclinical hypothyroidism and hypoadrenalism were suspected in 30 and 40 patients respectively. Superinfections associated with immune dysfunction [e.g., bowel parasites or yeast over-

growth] were suspected in 30 cases. Improvement with micronutrient supplementation was noted.

Depression, anxiety/hyperventilation and situational stresses
were considered to be the primary processes in 4, 4, and 3
patients respectively.

Treatment resulted in complete resolution of fatigue in 57%
and significant but incomplete improvement in 39% of the
patients. Improvement was seen at a median time of seven weeks.

Conclusions: Severe chronic fatigue states are multifactorial
processes that, in many patients, respond well to treatment.
*[Article copies available from The Haworth Document Delivery Service:
1-800-342-9678.]*

KEYWORDS. Fatigue, fibromyalgia, adrenal insufficiency, hypothyroidism, chronic fatigue syndrome

INTRODUCTION

Severe chronic fatigue states [SCFS] are common. Chronic
fatigue syndrome [CFS], representing a small subset of SCFS, is
rare. A recent report by Price et al. (1) suggests that only one in
13,535 people [or approximately 20,000 patients in the United
States] meet strict Center for Disease Control [CDC] criteria for
CFS. By CDC estimates, the prevalence is even lower, at 2-7 per
100,000 (2). The prevalence of persistent, often disabling, fatigue
has been estimated to be much higher—often up to six million
patients for fibromyalgia alone (3). Unfortunately, despite having
sought help for many years, people suffering from severe fatigue
often receive little benefit from treatment. This paper reports on
an approach to the evaluation and treatment of severe chronic
fatigue states which we have found to be effective.

A key factor in helping patients with chronic fatigue was the
realization that a combination of interrelated problems was usually
occurring. Patients often improved dramatically and quickly when
all the underlying problems were treated simultaneously. If only
one problem was treated, or if the problems were not treated
simultaneously, often the patient's improvement was only partial.
In our current study, we examined 64 patients with chronic and

severe fatigue to define the multiple underlying causes and to assess the efficacy of treating all the discovered problems.

MATERIALS AND METHODS

The study population consisted of 56 females and 8 males, ages 20 to 77 years [average age 45 years] whose major complaint was severe chronic fatigue of at least two month's duration which the patients felt significantly limited their activity. These patients were characterized by a mix of symptoms including recurrent upper respiratory infections [URIs], sore throats, swollen glands, increased thirst, achiness, poor sleep, and poor memory and concentration. We defined these patients as having a severe chronic fatigue state.

These patients presented in our office from 1991–1993. Most of these patients had been through numerous evaluations and/or treatments without relief before entering our trial. The median duration of their fatigue was 3 years [average 2 yrs; range 2 months–25 yrs]. Patients were given a thorough history and physical examination. Complete blood count [CBC], automated chemistry profile [Chem 19], erythrocyte sedimentation rate [ESR], urinalysis [UA], B12, serum iron, total iron binding capacity [TIBC], ferritin, glycosylated hemoglobin, thyroid functions and cortrosyn stimulation testing were done. In refractory cases, we checked for stool ova/parasites [O&P], Giardia and Cryptosporidium [tested in 19 patients]. Special attention was given to checking for:

1. Subclinical hypothyroidism—for the reasons noted in the discussion, if the free thyroxine [FT4] index was low normal and signs and symptoms suggestive of hypothyroidism were present [e.g. constipation, cold intolerance, low temperature, delayed ankle tendon relaxation phase, etc.], a low-dose Synthroid trial [25–50 mcg] was considered [especially if fibromyalgia was present]. If the thyroid stimulating hormone [TSH] was > 4 or < 0.8 [with a low normal FT4 index], this also weighed in favor of treatment. The free FT4 and ultrasensitive TSH assays are microparticle enzyme immunoassays for the quantitative determination of free thyroxine and human thyroid stimulating hormone in human serum as measured on Abbotts IMX.

2. Decreased Adrenal Function—A cortrosyn stimulation test was performed at 8:00 a.m. Fasting baseline, 30- and 60-minute serum cortisol levels were checked after a 25 unit dose of cortrosyn [ACTH] intramuscularly. The test was considered positive for a low baseline if the cortisol was < 6 mcg/dL. As our experience grew, we found patients often benefitted dramatically from treatment even if the baseline was as high as 11 mcg/dL. Therefore, we expanded our definition of low baseline to include patients with cortisol levels of up to 11 mcg/dL. These patients received a trial of treatment if they failed to respond fully to other treatment. If a patient showed low adrenal reserve [i.e., not doubling at one hour or not increasing by 7 mcg/dL at one-half hour and 11 mcg/dL by one hour], the patient was also treated. Although Jefferies (4,5) felt that most patients needed four times daily [q.i.d.] dosing of Cortef [e.g., Cortef 5 mg q.i.d.], we found that most of those with low reserve did well with 5 mg Cortef orally [p.o.] each morning [q.a.m.] and, if needed, 2.5 to 5 mg at lunchtime. Those with low baselines were more likely to need 5 to 7.5 mg three times daily [t.i.d.] or q.i.d. Those who don't respond to lower dosing should receive a trial of q.i.d. dosing [giving only 2.5 mg for the bedtime [q.h.s.] dose]. The cortisol assay is a homogeneous enzyme immunoassay for the quantitation of total cortisol in serum. The reagents are from Cedia Microgenics Corporation and run on the Technicon R.A.

3. Fibromyalgia—Diagnosis was made by the 1990 American College of Rheumatology tender point criteria. Amitriptyline [10–50 mg], cyclobenzaprine [5–20 mg], or Trazodone [25–75 mg] q.h.s. were used to treat disordered sleep in most fibromyalgia patients [see Table 3]. We use the terms Fibrositis and Fibromyalgia interchangeably.

4. Chronic infections

   A. Bacterial—Urinary tract infection [UTI], chronic sinusitis, or other infections were checked for by history and urinalysis. Most of these had been treated by other physicians before the patient's arrival in our office.

   B. Bowel parasites—Toward the end of our study, we tested patients refractory to other treatment for bowel parasites. The yield with routine O&P is low even if parasites are present. Because of this we used a purged stool specimen and had the slides read by our lab supervisor and a technologist experienced in looking for stool parasites. Antigen tests for Giardia and Cryptosporidium were also done. We now test all our chronic fatigue patients for bowel parasites. The objective of the stool purge was to secure a watery, "explosive" sample (6). We feel this gives far better reliability than numerous random samples. Patients are instructed to drink 1-1/2 ounces of Fleet Phospho-Soda and to collect the watery stool specimens in the three vials containing the preservative sodium acetate–acidic acid–formalin [SAF]. We use Meridian Diagnostic Para Pak SAF System and Para Pak Concentration Kit and trichrome stain for differentiation of internal structure of intestinal parasites.

C. Fungal infections—History was taken for risk factors suggestive of possible fungal overgrowth, e.g., frequent antibiotic use, recurrent vaginal or skin fungal infections, etc. If this raised a high index of suspicion or the stool microscopic examination was suggestive of fungal overgrowth, a trial of nystatin one million units p.o. q.i.d. was given over four to six months. We are currently finding itraconazole [taken with food] 200 mg p.o. daily [q.d.] for three to four weeks followed by 100 mg q.d. for one to four months in combination with Nystatin 500,000 units p.o. q.i.d. [while on itraconazole] to be more effective. Fluconazole may also be helpful in these patients. Nizoral may aggravate the often subtle adrenal insufficiency frequently seen in patients with chronic fatigue (7).

5. Depression, anxiety or hyperventilation—These were treated with tricyclic or selective serotonin reuptake inhibitors [SSRI] [e.g., Prozac] family of antidepressants if the symptoms were felt to have preceded the fatigue, as opposed to being caused by it. Patients who presented with an ongoing diagnosis of depression without other factors contributing to their fatigue were excluded from the study.

6. Possible micronutrient deficiencies—all patients were placed on a B complex [25 mg] vitamin with minerals [e.g., Berocca Plus or Twin Lab Daily One Caps]. Many were placed on Slow Mag [magnesium chloride] 2–6 tablets per day [less if diarrhea occurred]. Low iron and B12 were tested for and treated when present.

We felt that treating coexisting problems simultaneously would improve the effectiveness of treatment. Unfortunately this made it difficult to assess the degree of effectiveness of each individual treatment.

As the patient's symptoms in severe chronic fatigue states are predominately subjective, the determination of degree of improvement after any given treatment was made by the patient. This was complicated, at times, by several treatments being given concurrently.

The experimental nature of parts of the treatment was reviewed with the patient and informed consent was obtained.

RESULTS

As shown in Table 1, 37 of 64 patients had almost complete resolution of their fatigue and 25 of 64 showed significant, but incomplete, improvement. Two out of 64 patients had no significant improvement. Improvement was often rapid, at times occurring within a few days. Median length of symptoms before treatment was three years and median time to initial improvement was 1-3/4 months [i.e., first follow-up visit]. Patients did at times have temporary exacerbations during their treatment course. Improvement was, however, usually sustained [most patients have remained in follow-up for over one year]. Only seven patients had a single underlying contributing diagnosis. Most had three or four underlying problems [see Table 1]. Table 2 shows the number of patients felt to have each of the different underlying diagnoses and their response to treatment. Table 3 gives a more detailed breakdown of patient characteristics, contributing diagnoses, and responses to treatment.

DISCUSSION

We found that most patients [all but 7] had a combination of at least two underlying problems and 46 patients had more than two problems. Previous trials have often shown disappointing results when only one underlying cause was sought or treated.

TABLE 1. Clinical characteristics of the treatment group and the effect of treatment.

Number of patients	64
Male	8
Female	56

Ages	
Range	20–77 years old
Average	45 years old

Duration symptoms present	
Range	2 months to 25 years
Median	3 years
Average	2 years

Time until initial improvement was seen with treatment	
Range	4 days to 15 months
Average	3 months
Median	1.75 months [i.e., first follow-up visit]

Number of contributing diagnoses per patient	# of patients
1	7
2	11
3	23
4	13
5	9
6	0
7	1

Degree of improvement [out of 64 patients]	# of patients
Much improved [i.e., fatigue no longer a significant problem]	37
Moderate improvement [significant improvement but fatigue is still a problem]	25
No significant improvement	2

We found that patients—even those with fatigue of over 10 years duration—experienced [usually rapid] resolution of their symptoms 57% of the time and significant improvement another 39% of the time if the multiple underlying problems were identified and treated. Frankly, we were surprised at the degree of improvement shown by our patients.

Why did these patients show such an assortment of problems? The patterns we observed suggested that the primary process might have been hypothalamic dysfunction [caused by viral or

TABLE 2. Number of patients with each suspected diagnosis and response to treatment.

Suspected Diagnosis	Number of Patients	Improved with Treatment	No Clear Improvement with Rx	No Rx or Follow Up
A. Fibromyalgia	44	37	4	3
B. Low Thyroid				
1. By low T7/ high TSH	12	11	1	
2. By symptom/ exam only	18	14	3	1
C. Underactive Adrenal [Hypocortisolism]:				
1 Low adrenal baseline [i.e., 8 a.m Cortisol 0–5 9 mcg/dL]	7	5	2	
2. 8 a.m. Cortisol 6–11 mcg/dL	16	11	3	2
3. Low adrenal reserve	16	15	1	
D. Fungal Overgrowth	23	14	7	2
E Possible Low B12				
1. <300 PG/ml	7	7		
2. 301–540 PG/ml	19	17	1	1
F. Bowel Parasites: [in 19 pts. checked]				
Cryptosporidium	3	0	3	
Entameba	2	2		
Visceral Larva Migrans	1	1		
Tapeworm	1	1		
G. Depression - primary	4	4		
- secondary	4	4		
Anxiety/hyperventilation	4	3	1	

NOTE: Severe situational stress was felt to be the primary process in 3 patients and a secondary process in 5. Ferritins of 0–20 ng/ml and 21–40 ng/ml were seen in 7 and 6 patients, respectively. The effect of iron supplementation was not separately monitored.

other infections] with secondary multiple endocrine [and possibly immune] abnormalities. As Dr. Sternberg notes in her excellent editorial on hypoimmune fatigue states (8), and Dr. Behan and others note in their studies, hypothalamic-pituitary-adrenal [HPA] axis dysfunction appears to be common in chronic fatigue states (9,10,11,12,13). This can manifest as borderline or overt adrenal insufficiency and borderline or overt hypothyroidism. In their study on fibromyalgia, Neeck et al. (9) examined baseline and TRH stimulated thyroid function. Although most fibromyalgia patients had normal baseline thyroid functions, their response to TRH stimulation was significantly blunted. The increase of TSH and T4 after TRH stimulation was approximately 90% greater for TSH [$P < 0.05$] and over 800% greater for FT4 [$P < 0.05$] in controls than in fibromyalgia patients. This, combined with a clinical picture suggestive of hypothyroidism, suggests that our current testing misses subtle, but clinically significant, hypothyroidism in these patients. This problem is often accentuated by a low normal TSH [secondary to hypothalamic dysfunction]. The low TSH can further mislead the clinician into thinking thyroid function is adequate. Impairment of receptors for thyroid and adrenal hormones may also impact here. In light of this, an empiric trial of Synthroid 25–50 mcg/d often resulted in marked improvement. It is suggested that the adrenal insufficiency be treated first. Otherwise, the administration of Synthroid may accelerate the metabolic breakdown of the patient's cortisol, exacerbating the patient's symptoms. Interestingly, many of our patients exhibited marked polydipsia with normal blood sugars. This raised the possibility of a mild diabetes insipidus component, although that possibility was not formally tested. Bakheit and Behan also noted upregulation of hypothalamic serotonin receptors in postviral fatigue syndrome (11).

Patients with severe chronic fatigue states are sometimes found to exhibit immune dysfunction with associated recurrent and persistent infections. Infections like persistent bowel cryptosporidium or fungal overgrowth also suggest an immune-suppressed state. We suspect that the immunologic abnormalities may be secondary to adrenal dysfunction. Chronic severe fatigue, myalgias, arthralgias and neuropsychiatric changes are often associated with persistently elevated interferon levels

TABLE 3. Review of individual patient data.

Age	M/F	Hypothyroid Dx/Efct		Hypoadrenal* Dx/Efct		Fibrositis Dx/Efct TR = TRAGER		B12 Level pg/ml Efct		Yeast Suspct. Dx/Efct	
53	M	+	+	8.6	+						
27	F			+	+			348	+	+	No Rx
45	F										
33	F					+	−	540	+		
45	F	+	+	4.8	−	+	No Rx				
40	F	sc	+	5.7	++	+	+	484	+		
47	M			76	+	+	+ TR			+	− S.E
42	F	sc	+	+	+	+	+ TR				
44	F			7	++						
44	F									+	+
51	F	sc	+	+	++	+	+ TR				
53	F	+	+								
38	F					+	−	270	+		
53	F	+	+			+	+ TR				
33	F	sc	+			+	− S.E.W./Rx			+	+
37	F	sc	+	4.7	+	+	+			+	+
40	F	sc	+			+	+	440	+	+	+
50	F	sc	+	4	+	+	No Rx				
50	F					+	+ TR	300	+		
59	F										
34	F	+	+	3	−	+	+			+	+
30	F					+	+	294	+	+	+
41	F					+	+ TR				
26	M	sc	++	+	+	+	+				
55	F			1	++	+	+ TR				
73	F	+	+					220	+		
43	F			+	++	+	+				
42	F	+	+	+	±			524	+	+	−
31	F	sc	+	11	+	+	+	400	+	+	No Rx
29	F	sc	+	8	+	+	No Rx				
21	F	sc	±	+	+	+	+ TR				
51	F	sc	+	9	+	+	+			+	+
57	F	sc	+								

O & P	E F C T	Depressed Anxious Hyper-ventilatory	Ferritin	Symptoms present x mo/yrs	Time until improvement	Much better	Mod. better	No sig. chng.
				few months	1 month		+	
				2-1/2 years	6 weeks		+	
		work stress		1 year	15 months left	+		
				>1 year	4–6 months	+		
				app. 10 years	1 year	+		
				1 year	7 weeks	+		
				3-1/2 years	2-1/2 months	+		
		stress		9 months	3 months		+	
		stress		N/A	1 month	+		
				1 year	3 months	+		
				app. 4 months	2 months	+		
				2 months	<2 months		+	
		S.L.E.	28	5 years	1 year 2 months with B12		+	
				1-1/2 years	2 months		+	
				10 years	weeks	+		
				years	6 weeks	+		
				app. 2–3 months	2 months	+		
			29	N/A	6 weeks	+		
				4 years	N/A	+		
				years	without improvement			+
−				>6 years	months	+		
				2 years	1 month		+	
				>4 years	1 month	+		
				3 years	2 months		+	
		HV	23	years intermittent	2 months	+		
		depressed		months	<1 week	+		
				months	1–2 months	+		
			5	8–10 years	4 months		+	
		depressed	20	5 years	2 months		+	
				10 years	4–6 months	+		
				years	4 months		+	
		stress		1-1/2 years	N/A		+	
		depressed		years	4 months		+	

Age	M/F	Hypothyroid Dx/Efct		Hypoadrenal* Dx/Efct		Fibrositis Dx/Efct TR = TRAGER		B12 Level pg/ml Efct		Yeast Suspct. Dx/Efct	
67	F	sc	No Rx	9	No Rx	+	+				
20	F	sc	+	+	+			260	+		
51	F			11	+	+	+	247	+		
33	F	+	+					219	+		
57	F	+	+	+	+	+	+				
48	F			6	−	+	+	359	+	+	−
51	F					+	+	425	No Rx	+	+
40	F					+	+			+	±
39	F			11	− worse	+	+			+	+
49	M			6	−			323	−		
67	M										
58	F			+	++	+	−				
59	M					+	+	513	+	+	+
35	F				TR +	+	+ TR	340	+	+	−
34	F	sc	−	+	+	+	+				
39	F	sc	−	+	+	+	+			+	+
45	F			11	+	+	+				
34	F	+	+			+	+				
45	F			10	++	+	+ TR	425	+	+	+
40	F			2	+			340	+		
74	F					+	+	380	+		
77	M			8	+						
63	M			6	+						
46	F	+	+	+	++			328	+	+	±
44	F					+	+	371	+	+	−
45	F					+	+	387	+		
43	F			10	No Rx	+	++ TR				
43	F	sc	+	+	+	+	+	454	+		
41	F	+	−	+	+					+	+
31	F			+	+	+	+	206	+		
36	F									+	+

*Hypoadrenalism—If based on a low baseline cortisol, the baseline cortisol [in mcg/dl] is noted A [+] indicates an inadequate adrenal reserve [see Methods] EFCT = Effect of treatment. A [+] means the patient improved with treatment. A [−] means no improvement with treatment. SC = Subclinical. DX means patient had this diagnosis if [+] is in the column. CS = Cryptosporidium. VLM = Visceral larva migrans Ferritin is in ng/ml.

O & P	E F C T	Depressed Anxious Hyper-ventilatory	Ferritin	Symptoms present x mo/yrs	Time until improvement	Much better	Mod. better	No sig. chng.
				4–5 years	2 months	+		
				months	1–2 months	+		
		depressed	21	>4 years	4 months	+		
			20	1 year	2 months		+	
				years inter.	4 months	+		
		anxious		>20 years	5 months	+		
CS	–	anxious depressed	30	years	1 week after Sporanox		+	
				6 years	6 weeks	+		
CS	–	depressed		7 years	7 months		+	
		depressed		years	N/A			+
		depressed		6 years	10 months	+		
				many years	2 months	+		
				5–6 years	3 months		+	
				4 years	2 months		+	
				N/A	N/A		+	
				years	2 months		+	
VLM	+	stress		1 year	6 weeks		+	
				1–2 years	1 month	+		
			3	9 years	3 months	+		
			26	1-1/2 years	2 weeks	+		
Tape Worm	+			years	months		+	
CS	–	stress		4 months	2 months	+		
				1 year	3 months	+		
				8 months	2 months	+		
		H V.	14	2 years	6 weeks		+	
Entmba +	+		19	15 years	1 month	+		
				years	1 month	+		
				25 years	2 months	+		
				2 years	1–2 months		+	
Entmba+			46	4 years	4 days	+		
		stress	18	2–3 years	N/A		+	

(14,15). Cortisol also lowers interferon levels (16). Interestingly, metoclopramide and naloxone have been reported to improve interferon induced fatigue (14,15), although we've not tried these medications. It would be interesting to test interferon levels before and after treatment with cortisol and see if levels correlate with symptomatic improvement, as elevated interferon can mimic or cause many of the symptoms and signs [e.g., achiness, muscle mitochondrial changes and fatigue] seen in chronic fatigue patients (14,15). This could offer another mechanism for cortisol's effectiveness. Other adrenal androgens [e.g., testosterone, dehydroepiandrosterone [DHEA] and DHEA-S] also have significant effects on lymphokine production (16) and lower levels in females could explain their increased susceptibility. We recently tested DHEA-S levels in three patients with abnormal cortrosyn tests and found DHEA-S levels to be very low. ACTH is widely accepted as a regulating factor for adrenal androgen secretion under certain conditions (16). Further studies of interleukin [IL] 2, 4, and 5 function in these patients would help define the immune dysfunction further. DHEA, for example, increases IL-2 and gamma-interferon [gamma-IFN]. Testosterone decreases IL-4, IL-5 and gamma-IFN. Glucocorticoids inhibit gamma-IFN and IL-2 (16). Although the cause of the immune dysfunction is not clear, the above suggest possible mechanisms by which hypothalamic suppression could be involved.

Jefferies (4,5) noted several decades ago that severe fatigue and recurrent URIs following a severe viral infection were often caused by adrenal insufficiency and resolved with cortisol treatment. He theorized that the fatigue was caused by a transient, and at times permanent, inhibition of ACTH production by the viral infection. This theory was recently supported by the work of Demitrack and Dale (10). In several thousand patient years of experience, Jefferies found these patients improved dramatically on low-dose cortisol. There was no toxicity [except mild gastritis] as long as the dosage was physiologic [e.g., 5 mg t.i.d. to q.i.d. of cortisol] and not pharmacologic (4,5). Our findings support Jefferies' experience. Patients with low adrenal reserve [e.g., no doubling in one hour] usually did well with cortisol 5 mg q.a.m. and, if needed, 2.5 mg at lunch. Patients with low baselines were more likely to need cortisol 5–7.5 mg t.i.d. to q.i.d. [up to 30 mg/d with morning doses being higher]. Dr. Jefferies recommends that any patient who does not respond to b.i.d. dosing be given a trial of cortisol 2.5 to 5 mg p.o. q.i.d. Patients with reactive hypoglycemia were likely to be hypoadrenal, as cortisol helps to maintain blood glucose levels.

Although at times they are secondary to the immune or other dysfunctions, the fibromyalgia and the parasitic, bacterial, and fungal infections need to be treated as well or the patient's fatigue will persist. Fibromyalgia appears to be a common endpoint of many physical, physiologic, and/or psychological stress states. We view it as predominately a sleep disorder. These patients have multiple tender points and occasionally muscle trigger points which could interfere with deep sleep. These patients tend to toss and turn a lot at night and remain in light sleep stages. The quality of the deep sleep stages that "recharge their batteries" appears to be disordered. Thus, despite many hours of sleep, these patients can be considered to have not [effectively] slept for many years. The stress of sleeping ineffectively leaves the patient functioning poorly and may alter the HPA axis (13). This stress can aggravate the tender points and thus, the cycle continues. Treatment needs to be geared toward restoring the duration, and/or quality, of deep-stage sleep and resolving the patient's trigger and tender points.

Dr. Janet Travell, the personal physician to Presidents Kennedy and Johnson, is also one of the world's foremost experts on myofascial pain. In the *Trigger Point Manual*, Dr. Travell's and Dr. David Simon's book on myofascial pain (17), there is an excellent chapter on perpetuating factors that must be treated. Our experience suggests that the perpetuating factors in myofascial pain syndrome and fibromyalgia are similar. We have found the a mix of therapies will usually cause fibromyalgia to improve or fully resolve. Our regimen consists of: A. Treatment with amitriptyline 10–50 mg/h.s. or trazodone 25–150 mg/h.s. or cyclobenzaprine 5–10 mg/h.s. B. Nutritional support, e.g., Berocca Plus [or Twin Lab Daily One Cap] vitamins one a day long term plus Slow Mag [magnesium chloride] 2 tabs t.i.d. × 6 months. Correcting low Vitamin B12 and iron levels is important. C. It is important to treat even borderline hypothyroidism and hypoadrenalism [as discussed previously]. D. Exercise [when the patient starts to improve]. E. For our refractory patients, we've found a form of neuromuscular reeducation [Trager—per Milton Trager, M.D.] to be very beneficial. F. Correcting structural perpetuating factors such as uneven leg lengths, small hemipelvis, short upper arms [adjust chair arms], etc., is important. G. As noted below it is also important to treat any occult underlying infections.

Chronic fatigue patients often have a mix of underlying infections caused by [and perhaps aggravating] their immune dysfunction. We found that treating these was critical. Most patients had a marked decrease in their recurrent viral infections on cortisol. Chronic sinusitis, UTI, and other bacterial infections are readily detectable. Bowel yeast overgrowth is harder to test for and, therefore, we considered treating the patient empirically if they had frequent antibiotic use or frequent vaginal or dermatologic fungal infections [i.e., suggestive of increased risk of or a decreased resistance to fungal infections]. We used Nystatin 1 million units p.o. q.i.d. in this study. Our current experience suggests that adding itraconazole [Sporanox] 200 mg p.o. q.d. with food for three to four weeks followed by 100 mg p.o. q.d. [to the Nystatin] may be more effective. Bowel parasites also needed to be treated and were surprisingly common [7 of 19 patients tested]. Samples should be obtained after a Phospho-Soda laxative (6) and tested for in a lab familiar with parasite detection [see methods]. Otherwise, the low sensitivity will make this an unreliable test.

In many patients, the above problems appear to be associated with increased nutritional needs. Many patients with only mild to moderate fatigue [and therefore not included in this series] have their symptoms resolve fully, simply by taking a Twin Lab Daily One Cap vitamin or Berocca Plus q.d. and Slow-Mag [magnesium as the chloride—67 mg] 2 t.i.d. and avoiding excess sugar, caffeine, and alcohol. This is an important part of the regimen for the severely fatigued patient in our current series as well.

Lindenbaum et al. (18) found that barely subnormal or occasionally even normal B12 levels can be associated with evidence of severe neuropsychiatric changes caused by cobalamin deficiency—even in the absence of anemia or macrocytosis. These included memory loss, fatigue, and personality changes. Similar findings were noted by Carmel (19). Norman (20) also noted that as many as 40% of B12-deficient individuals may have been missed by simply relying on serum B12 levels. These were found by checking urine methylmalonic acid. Lindenbaum et al.'s recent study confirms that B12 deficiency can occur even with vitamin B12 levels over 500 PG/ml (21). Because the level at which neuropsychiatric changes cease to occur is not well defined, a trial of B12 1 mg IM q. week for eight weeks was given in some patients with levels of up to 540 PG/ml to rule out subclinical B12 deficiency. Surprisingly, 24 of 26 patients had significant improvement. Some patients benefit from continuing with B12 injections 1 mg IM q. 3–5 weeks. Most others did not need this after the initial series of injections. A trial of iron treatment was also considered if ferritin levels were less than 40 ng/ml.

As in any other illness, psychological factors, including depression, anxiety, and psychological conflicts, are critical here and must be addressed. We found that lack of interests correlated well with depression being primary [found in only 4/64 patients]. If the patient had many interests, but was frustrated over not having the energy to fulfill them, the depression was usually considered to be secondary to the fatigue. This is corroborated by the common finding of high baseline cortisols in patients whose depression is primary. The frequency of low morning cortisol levels makes it unlikely that endogenous depression is common in chronic fatigue state patients (12).

Patients may at times have intermittent exacerbations of their symptoms while physical and psychological issues are being worked through. Recurrence of previous problems [e.g., low B12 or infections] occasionally occurs and requires retreatment. Continuing to guide and assist patients through this period is very important. Doing this, we have found that most patients maintained their improvement during the one to two year poststudy period.

Initially, we considered limiting the study to patients who met strict CFS [chronic fatigue syndrome] criteria. Recent reports, however, suggest that immunologic abnormalities seen in CFS patients [vs. controls] are no different than those seen in other patients with severe fatigue (22). Our experience also suggested that the underlying causes and the response to treatment were not affected by whether patients strictly met criteria for CFS. Because of these two reasons, we elected to study all patients who found their fatigue to be severe and persistent and whose constellation of symptoms was similar to CFS, even if they did not fulfill all of the criteria for CFS.

Ideally, we would have liked to have done a controlled cross-over study for all variables and to test the effect of each treatment separately. Simultaneous treatment of the patient's underlying problems may be required, however, to cause the symptoms to resolve. We therefore chose, instead, to begin with an open clinical trial. At this point, we are planning a future controlled trial. Areas that would be good candidates for a controlled study within the above context would include: 1. low-dose cortisol for patients with borderline low cortrosyn test baselines [Cortisol of 6 to 13 mcg/dL] or borderline low adrenal reserve values; 2. A trial of itraconazole or fluconazole vs. placebo in patients with recurrent fungal infections; 3. B12 injections as above vs. placebo for patients with B12 levels of 208–540 PG/ml. The controlled trial may also decrease the problem of defining clearly which treatments are causing the improvement, as several treatments were often begun simultaneously.

Much of our experience confirms the old adage that "even a blind squirrel finds acorns." We are certain that there is much more to learn in this area. In the interim, it is hoped that the above report creates new avenues to explore in understanding the treatment of severe chronic fatigue.

REFERENCES

1.   Price RK, North CS, Nessely S, Fraser, VJ: Estimating the prevalence of chronic fatigue syndrome in the community. Public Health Reports 107: 514–22, Sept–Oct 1992.

2.   Marchesani RB: Critical antiviral pathway deficient in CFS patients. Infectious Disease News 4, August 1993.

3.   Goldenberg DL: Fibromyalgia syndrome. JAMA 257: 2782–87, 1987.

4.   Jefferies W: Safe Uses of Cortisone. Charles C. Thomas [Publisher], Springfield, 1981.

5. Jefferies W: Low dose glucocorticoid therapy. Archives of Internal Medicine 119: 265–78, 1967.

6. Rosenbaum M, Susser M: Solving the Puzzle of Chronic Fatigue Syndrome. Life Sciences Press, Tacoma, 1992.

7. Medical Letter: 34: 14, Feb 1992.

8. Sternberg EM: Hypoimmune fatigue syndromes—Diseases of the stress response. [Editorial] J Rheumatol 20: 418–21, 1993.

9. Neeck G, Riedel W: Thyroid function in patients with fibromyalgia syndrome. J Rheumatol 19: 1120–22, 1992.

10. Demitrack MA, Dale JK, Strauss SE, Laue L, Listwak SJ, Kruesi, MJ: Evidence for impaired activation of the hypothalamic-pituitary-adrenal axis in patients with chronic fatigue syndrome. J Clin Endo Metab 73: 1224–34, 1991.

11. Bakheit Amo, Behan PO, Dinan TG, Gray, CE, O'Keane V: Possible upregulation of hypothalamic 5HT receptors in patients with postviral fatigue syndrome. BMJ 304: 1010–12, April 1992.

12. Griep EN, Boersma JW, deKlset ER: Altered reactivity of the HPA axis in the primary fibromyalgia syndrome. J Rheumatol 20: 469–474, 1993.

13. McCain GA, Tilbe KS: Diurnal hormone variation in fibromyalgia syndrome: A comparison with Rheumatoid Arthritis. J Rheumatol 25: 469–474, 1993.

14. Quesada JR, Talpaz M, Rios A, Kurzrock R, Gutterman JU: Clinical toxicity of interferons in cancer patients: A review. J Clin Oncology 4: 234–43, Feb 1986.

15. Adams F, Quesada JR, Gutterman JU: Neuropsychiatric manifestations of human leucocyte interferon therapy in patients with cancer. JAMA 252: 938–941, 1984.

16. Meikle AW, Daynes RA, Araneo BA, Parker LN: Adrenal androgen secretion and biologic effects and control of adrenal androgen secretion. Endocrine and Metab. Clinics of North America 20, #2: 381–421, June 1991.

17. Travell JG, Simons DG: Myofascial Pain & Dysfunction; The Trigger Point Manual. Williams & Wilkins, Baltimore, 1983, pp. 103–64.

18. Lindenbaum J, Healton EB, Savage DG, Brust JCM, Garrett TJ, Podell ER: Neuropsychiatric disorders caused by cobalamin deficiency in the absence of anemia or macrocytosis. NEJM 318: 1720–28, 1988.

19.   Carmel R: Pernicious Anemia—The expected findings of very low serum cobalamin levels, anemia and macrocytosis are often lacking. Arch Intern Med 148: 1712–14, 1988.

20.   Norman EJ, Morrison JA: Screening for Vitamin B12 deficiency using urinary MMA. Am J Med 94: 589–94, June 1993.

21.   Lindenbaum J, Rosenberg IH, Wilson PWF, Stabler SP, Allen RH: Prevalence of cobalamin deficiency in the Framingham elderly population. Am J Clin Nutr 60: 2–11, 1994.

22.   Strauss SE, Fritz S, Dale JK, Gould B, Strober W: Lymphocyte phenotype and function in CFS. J Clin Immunol 13: 30–40, Jan 1993.

Originally published in the *Journal of Musculoskeletal Pain* 3 (1995). 91–110. Used courtesy of Haworth Press

Appendix C

Recommended Reading

BOOKS

Ali, M. *The Canary and Chronic Fatigue*. Denville, NJ: IPM Press, 1994. Focuses on the damage to enzyme systems by environmental stresses and nutritional-herbal-lifestyle therapeutics.

Bell, D. S. *Curing Fatigue*. Emmaus, PA: Rodale Press, 1993. Includes good common-sense approaches to fatigue.

Crook, W. G. *Chronic Fatigue Syndrome and the Yeast Connection*. Jackson, TN: Professional Books, 1992.

Crook, W. G. *The Yeast Connection*. Jackson, TN: Professional Books, 1983. Gives an overview of problems believed to be caused by yeast overgrowth. Out of print.

Crook, W. G. *The Yeast Connection and the Woman*. Jackson, TN: Professional Books, 1995. An excellent book.

Dawson, D. M., and T. D. Sabin. *Chronic Fatigue Syndrome*. Boston, MA: Little, Brown and Co., 1993. An overview for physicians.

Forman, R. *How to Control Your Allergies*. Atlanta, GA: Larchmont Books, 1979. Diagnosis and treatment of food allergies.

Goldstein, J. *Betrayal by the Brain: The Neurologic Basis of Chronic Fatigue Syndrome, Fibromyalgia Syndrome and Related Neural Network Disorders*. Binghampton, NY: Haworth Press, 1996.

Goldstein, J. *Treatment Options in Chronic Fatigue Syndrome: A Guide for Physicians and Patients*. Binghampton, NY: Haworth Press, 1995.

Hyde, B. M. *The Clinical and Scientific Bases of Myalgic Encephalitis and Chronic Fatigue Syndrome*. Ottawa, ON: Nightingale Research Foundation, 1992. An encyclopedic review of CFS research.

Ivker, R. S. *Sinus Survival*. New York, NY: J. P. Tarcher, 1991. "Must reading" for patients with chronic sinusitis.

Jeffries, W. M. *Safe Uses of Cortisone*. Springfield, IL: Charles C. Thomas, 1981. A landmark monograph on adrenal insufficiency. Written for physicians.

Rogers, S. A. *Tired or Toxic*. Syracuse, NY: Prestige Publishing, 1990. An extensive review of chemical sensitivity problems.

Rosenbaum, M., and M. Susser. *Solving the Puzzle of Chronic Fatigue Syndrome*. Tacoma, WA: Life Sciences Press, 1992. A good review of CFS treatments and also of infectious problems.

Travell, J. G., and D. G. Simons. *Myofascial Pain and Dysfunction: The Trigger Point Manual*. Baltimore, MD: Williams & Wilkins, 1983. A crucial text for anyone treating myofascial (muscle) pain. Chapter 4 discusses perpetuating factors, which are also important when treating fibromyalgia.

JOURNALS

The CFIDS Chronicle. Chronic Fatigue and Immune Dysfunction Syndrome Association of America, P.O. Box 220398, Charlotte, NC 28222-0398. A subscription comes with membership in the Chronic Fatigue and Immune Dysfunction Syndrome Association of America.

The Journal of Chronic Fatigue Syndrome. Haworth Press, 10 Alice Street, Binghamton, NY 13904. For physicians.

The Journal of Musculoskeletal Pain. Haworth Press, 10 Alice Street, Binghamton, NY 13904. For physicians.

Appendix D

Yeast Questionnaire

Section A of this questionnaire lists aspects of your medical history that may promote growth of the common yeast *Candida albicans* and result in yeast-associated illness.

Sections B and C evaluate the presence of symptoms that are often found in individuals who suffer from yeast-connected illnesses.

For each "yes" answer in Section A, circle the point score. Total the points and record the score at the end of the section. Next, go to Sections B and C and score as directed.

SECTION A: YOUR MEDICAL HISTORY

		Point Score
1.	Have you been treated for acne with tetracycline, erythromycin, or any other antibiotic for one month or longer?	50
2.	Have you taken antibiotics for any type of infection for more than two consecutive months, or in shorter courses four or more times in any twelve-month period?	50
3.	Have you ever taken an antibiotic—even for a single course?	6
4.	Have you ever had prostatitis, vaginitis, or another infection or problem with your reproductive organs for more than one month?	25

		Point Score
5.	Have you been pregnant:	
	Two or more times?	5
	Once?	3
6.	Have you taken birth control pills for:	
	More than two years?	15
	Six months to two years?	8
7.	Have you taken a corticosteroid such as prednisone, Cortef, or Medrol by mouth or inhaler for:	
	More than two weeks?	15
	Two weeks or less?	6
8.	When you are exposed to perfumes, insecticides, or other odors or chemicals, do you develop wheezing, burning eyes, or any other distress?	
	Yes, and the symptoms keep me from continuing my activities.	20
	Yes, but the symptoms are mild and do not change my activities.	5
9.	Are your symptoms worse on damp or humid days or in moldy places?	20
10.	Have you ever had a fungal infection, such as jock itch, athlete's foot, or a nail or skin infection, that was difficult to treat and:	
	Lasted more than two months?	20
	Lasted less than two months?	10
11.	Do you crave:	
	Sugar?	10
	Breads?	10
	Alcoholic beverages?	10
12.	Does tobacco smoke cause you discomfort such as wheezing, burning eyes, or another problem?	10

Total Score Section A

SECTION B: MAJOR SYMPTOMS

For each symptom that is present, enter the appropriate figure in the point score column:

If a symptom is occasional or mild . . . . Score 3 points.
If a symptom is frequent and/or
    moderately severe . . . . Score 6 points.
If a symptom is severe and/or disabling . . . . . . Score 9 points.

Add the total score for this section and record it at the end of the section.

                                                        Point Score

1. Fatigue or lethargy.   _____

2. Feeling of being "drained."   _____

3. Poor memory.   _____

4. Feeling "spacey" or "unreal."   _____

5. Inability to make decisions.   _____

6. Numbness, burning, or tingling.   _____

7. Insomnia.   _____

8. Muscle aches.   _____

9. Muscle weakness or paralysis.   _____

10. Pain and/or swelling in joints.   _____

11. Abdominal pain.   _____

12. Constipation.   _____

13. Diarrhea.   _____

14. Bloating, belching or intestinal gas.   _____

15. Troublesome vaginal burning, itching,
    or discharge.   _____

16. Prostatitis.   _____

17. Impotence.   _____

18. Loss of sexual desire or feeling.   _____

Point Score

19. Endometriosis or infertility.   _____

20. Cramps and/or other menstrual irregularities.   _____

21. Premenstrual tension.   _____

22. Attacks of anxiety or crying.   _____

23. Cold hands or feet and/or chilliness.   _____

24. Shaking or irritable when hungry.   _____

Total Score Section B   _____

SECTION C: OTHER SYMPTOMS*

For each symptom that is present, enter the appropriate figure in the point score column:

If a symptom is occasional or mild . . . . Score 1 point.
If a symptom is frequent and/or
   moderately severe . . . . Score 2 points.
If a symptom is severe and/or persistent . . . . . . Score 3 points.

   Add the total score for this section and record it at the end of the section.

Point Score

1. Drowsiness.   _____

2. Irritability or jitteriness.   _____

3. Incoordination.   _____

4. Inability to concentrate.   _____

5. Frequent mood swings.   _____

6. Headache.   _____

7. Dizziness, loss of balance.   _____

8. Pressure above ears, feeling of head swelling. _____

*While the symptoms in this section occur commonly in patients with yeast-connected illness, they also occur commonly in patients who do not have Candida

Point Score

9. Tendency to bruise easily. _____

10. Chronic rashes or itching. _____

11. Psoriasis or recurrent hives. _____

12. Indigestion or heartburn. _____

13. Food sensitivity or intolerance. _____

14. Mucus in stools. _____

15. Rectal itching. _____

16. Dry mouth or throat. _____

17. Rash or blisters in mouth. _____

18. Bad breath. _____

19. Foot, hair, or body odor not relieved by washing. _____

20. Nasal congestion or postnasal drip. _____

21. Nasal itching. _____

22. Sore throat. _____

23. Laryngitis, loss of voice. _____

24. Cough or recurrent bronchitis. _____

25. Pain or tightness in chest. _____

26. Wheezing or shortness of breath. _____

27. Urinary frequency, urgency, or incontinence. _____

28. Burning on urination. _____

29. Spots in front of eyes or erratic vision. _____

30. Burning or tearing of eyes. _____

31. Recurrent infections or fluid in ears. _____

32. Ear pain or deafness. _____

Total Score Section C _____

Total Score Section B _____

Total Score Section A _____

Grand Total Score (Add up Total Scores from Sections A, B, and C) _____

The Grand Total Score will help you and your physician decide if your health problems are yeast-connected. Scores in women will run higher, as seven items in the questionnaire apply exclusively to them, while only two apply exclusively to men.

Yeast-connected health problems are almost certainly present in women with scores *over 160* and in men with scores *over 140*.

Yeast-connected health problems are probably present in women with scores *over 120* and in men with scores *over 90*.

Yeast-connected health problems are possibly present in women with scores *over 60* and in men with scores *over 40*.

With scores of *less than 60* in women and *40* in men, yeasts are less apt to be the cause of health problems.

Adapted from W. G Crook, M.D., *The Yeast Connection and the Woman* (Jackson, TN: Professional Books, 1995) and *The Yeast Connection Handbook* (Jackson, TN: Professional Books, 1996). Used with permission.

Appendix E

Fibromyalgia Information Questionnaire

1. How long have you been fatigued?_____

   How much has fatigue decreased your functioning? _____
   _____

2. Was the onset of your illness sudden or gradual?_____
   _____

3. If it was sudden:

   a. What was the date of onset? _____

   b. What symptoms presented at onset?_____

4. What stresses did you have in your life when the disease began?_____
   _____
   _____

5. Did your symptoms begin soon or immediately after a pregnancy? Describe._____
   _____
   _____

6. How many children do you have?_____

   What are their ages? _____

7. Are you married, single, divorced, or widowed? _____

   If you are married, for how long? _____

   What is your spouse's name? _____

   Is your spouse supportive of you? _____

8. How many hours per week were you working (aside from caring for your family) at the onset of your illness? _____

   _____

   How many hours per week do you work now? _____

   _____

9. What is your occupation? _____

10. Did you have to change jobs or decrease how much you work because of your illness? If yes, please describe.

    _____

    _____

    _____

11. Do you have any family members with fibromyalgia/chronic fatigue syndrome? _____

    If yes, how are they related to you and what are their ages? _____

    _____

12. What is your age?_____Date of birth? _____

13. Are you male or female? _____

14. How many doctors have you seen for your symptoms?

    _____

15. What other diagnoses/problems do you have? _____

    _____

16. What treatments are you on?
    a. Prescription_____

    b. Nonprescription_____

17. What treatments have you found helpful in the past? _____

    _____

18. What treatments have you tried without benefit? _____

    _____

19. What treatments have made you feel worse in the past? __

    _____

Symptom Checklist

Answer the following questions by circling Y for yes or N for no.

I. CFIDS CRITERIA

Y N   Is your fatigue *not* lifelong, is it *not* the result of
        ongoing exertion, is it *not* substantially alleviated by
        rest, and has it substantially reduced your partici-
        pation in occupational, educational, social, or
        personal activities?

Y N   Do you have four or more of the following symptoms?
        To apply, the symptom must have persisted or
        recurred during six or more consecutive months of
        illness and must not predate the fatigue. Circle the
        letter of each symptom that applies.

    A. Self-reported impairment of short-term memory
        or concentration that is severe enough to have
        caused a substantial reduction in your partici-
        pation in occupational, educational, social, or
        personal activities.

    B. Sore throat.

    C. Tender neck or axillary (armpit) lymph nodes.

    D. Muscle pain.

    E. Multijoint pain without joint swelling or redness.

    F. Headaches of a new type, pattern, or severity.

    G. Unrefreshing sleep.

H. Post-exertional fatigue lasting for more than twenty-four hours.

II. FIBROMYALGIA CRITERIA

Y   N   Have you had chronic widespread pain for more than three months in all four quadrants of your body (above and below your waist and on both sides of your body)? Have you also had axial pain (pain around your spine or chest)?

Y   N   When you exercise, do you feel worse afterwards and exhausted the next day?

Check off which of the following symptoms you have. (Several symptoms appear in more than one group.)

Adrenal Gland

_____   1. Hypoglycemia.
_____   2. Cravings for sweets.
_____   3. Shakiness relieved by eating.
_____   4. Dizziness.
_____   5. Moodiness.
_____   6. Recurrent infections that take a long time to resolve.
_____   7. A lot of stress in your life before your symptoms began.
_____   8. Low blood pressure.
_____   9. Dizziness upon first standing.
_____   10. Food cravings or sensitivities. Circle which ones and list the foods.

Thyroid Gland

_____   11. Weight gain. How much?_____ In what time period?_____
_____   12. Low body temperature (below 98°F).
_____   13. Constipation.
_____   14. Achiness.
_____   15. High cholesterol.
_____   16. Cold intolerance.

_____ 17. Dry skin.
_____ 18. Thin hair.
_____ 19. Heavy periods (females only).
_____ 20. Premenstrual syndrome (females only).
Describe symptoms. _____

_____

Other Hormones

_____ 21. Menopausal symptoms (females only).
_____ 22. Cold extremities.
_____ 23. Pallor (pale face).
_____ 24. Irregular periods (females only).
_____ 25. Decreased libido.
_____ 26. Decreased hair growth on arms or legs.
_____ 27. Delayed orgasm.
_____ 28. Decreased erections (males only).
_____ 29. One or both ovaries removed (females only).
_____ 30. Day or night sweats or hot flashes (females only).
_____ 31. Nipple discharge.

Vasopressor Syncope (NMH)

_____ 32. Low blood pressure.
_____ 33. Dizziness or disequilibrium. Circle which ones.
_____ 34. Increased thirst.

Lyme Disease

_____ 35. History of frequent tick bites. Describe how
many and where._____

_____

_____ 36. Rash following a tick bite.
_____ 37. Treatment for Lyme disease.
_____ 38. Numbness or tingling in fingers or feet.

Prostatitis (Males only)

_____ 39. Burning upon urination.
_____ 40. Aching groin.

_____ 41. Discharge from penis.
_____ 42. Urgent need to urinate but small output.

Sinusitis/Nasal Congestion

_____ 43. Chronic nasal congestion or postnasal drip.
_____ 44. Chronic yellow or green nasal discharge.
_____ 45. Chronic bad taste in mouth or bad breath.
_____ 46. Headaches under or over eyes.
_____ 47. Scratchy or watery eyes.

Disordered Sleep

_____ 48. Difficulty falling asleep.
_____ 49. Difficulty staying asleep.
_____ 50. Tendency to awaken during the night. Describe how often._____
_____ 51. Tendency to feel worse after exercise on same day or next day. Circle which ones.
_____ 52. Tendency to awaken at night due to need to urinate.

Yeast Overgrowth

_____ 53. Yeast infections (females only). Describe how often. _____
_____ 54. Fungal infections in toenails or fingernails.
_____ 55. Skin fungal infections (such as athlete's foot, jock itch, rash under bra.)
_____ 56. Frequent antibiotic use. Describe how often.
_____
_____ 57. Use of antibiotics for acne or prostatitis. Circle which ones.
_____ 58. Sugar cravings.
_____ 59. Bread cravings.
_____ 60. Frequent sores in the mouth.
_____ 61. Tendency toward cold sores or herpes attacks before or during symptom flare-up.

_____ 62. Prednisone use.

_____ 63. Use of birth control pills.

Parasites

_____ 64. Symptoms began with a diarrhea attack.

_____ 65. Diarrhea. Describe severity. _____

_____ 66. Constipation.

_____ 67. Bloating or increased gas.

_____ 68. Use of well water.

_____ 69. Abdominal cramps or gas.

Other Problems

_____ 70. Brain fog (poor memory or concentration).

_____ 71. Sensitivity to medications.

_____ 72. Chemical sensitivity.

_____ 73. Food intolerances. List foods. _____
_____

_____ 74. Use of nondiet sodas. Estimate daily intake.
_____

_____ 75. Use of coffee. Estimate how many eight-ounce
cups of regular and decaffeinated coffee you
drink per day. _____

_____ 76. Use of alcohol. Estimate daily intake. _____

_____ 77. Inability to exercise.

_____ 78. Stress. Describe._____
_____

_____ 79. Unusual weight gain or loss. How much? _____
In what time period? _____

_____ 80. Rashes. Describe._____

_____ 81. Chest pain, shortness of breath, or wheezing.
Circle which ones.

_____ 82. Palpitations or ankle swelling. Circle which ones.

_____ 83. Tendency to snore or stop breathing while
sleeping. Circle which ones.

_____ 84. Numbness or tingling around lips or mouth.

_____ 85. Panic attacks.

_____   86. Sudden inability to take a deep-enough breath
              or shortness of breath. Circle which ones.

_____   87. History of psychiatric illness. Describe.
              _____

_____   88. Depression (as opposed to frustration over not
              being able to function).

_____   89. Feelings of worthlessness, thoughts of suicide,
              low interest in most activities. Circle which
              ones.

_____   90. Other symptoms or problems. Describe.
              _____
              _____
              _____
              _____

Appendix F

Treatment Protocol for Chronic Fatigue Syndrome and Fibromyalgia

Dear Patient,

Following are the more common treatments for chronic fatigue syndrome and fibromyalgia. *Start them slowly!* For descriptions of these agents, see Information on Commonly Used Treatments for Chronic Fatigue Syndrome and Fibromyalgia.

NUTRITIONAL TREATMENTS

_____ 1. TwinLab Daily One Caps with or without iron, one every morning. Take with food if it upsets your stomach.

_____ 2. Magnesium chloride or lactate, two tablets three times a day for eight months, then two tablets once a day. Begin with one tablet a day and slowly increase the dose. Reduce the dose if diarrhea becomes a problem.

_____ 3. Fibrocare or Supermalic, two tablets two or three times a day for eight months, then two to four tablets once a day. Reduce the dose if diarrhea becomes a problem.

_____ 4. L-carnitine, 1,000 milligrams three times a day.

_____ 5. Coenzyme Q_{10},_____ milligrams _____ times a day.

_____ 6. Calcium, 500 to 1,000 milligrams a day. We recommend a chewable calcium or Os-Cal or Caltrate.

_____ 7. Ferrous-Sequels (iron), one tablet _____ times a day. Do not take within six hours of any hormone preparation, as this can prevent absorption.

_____ 8. Chromagen (iron), one tablet _____ times a day. Do not take within six hours of any hormone preparation, as this can prevent absorption.

_____ 9. Vitamin B_{12}, 1,000 micrograms, one shot once a week for _____ weeks.

_____ 10. Magnesium-potassium aspartate, 1,000 milligrams, two capsules one to two times a day.

SLEEPING AIDS FOR FIBROMYALGIA

_____ 1. Elavil, 10 milligrams, one-half to five at bedtime.

_____ 2. Flexeril, 10 milligrams, one-half to two at bedtime.

_____ 3. Desyrel, 50 milligrams, one-half to three at bedtime.

_____ 4. Ambien, 10 milligrams, one-half to two at bedtime.

_____ 5. Super Snooze (herbal sleep remedy), one to three at bedtime.

_____ 6. Valerian root (herbal sleep remedy), 360 to 450 milligrams, one at bedtime.

_____ 7. Lemon balm, 80 to 160 milligrams, plus valerian root, 180 to 360 milligrams, at bedtime. This combination is available as Valerian Rest (herbal sleep remedy).

_____ 8. Melatonin, .3 milligram, one at bedtime.

_____ 9. Klonopin, .5 milligram, one-half to four at bedtime. Begin with one-half tablet at bedtime and slowly increase the dose.

_____ 10. Soma, 350 milligrams, one-half to one at bedtime.

HORMONAL TREATMENTS

_____ 1. Synthroid, _____ micrograms, one every morning. Do not take within six hours of any iron preparation (except a multivitamin with iron), as this can prevent absorption.

_____ 2. Armour Thyroid, _____ grain, _____ tablets every morning.

_____ 3. Cortef, 5 milligrams, _____ tablets with breakfast, _____ tablets with lunch, and _____ tablets at 4 P.M.

_____ 4. DHEA, _____ milligrams every morning.

_____ 5. Florinef, .1 milligram, one every morning. Begin with one-quarter tablet every morning and increase by one-quarter tablet every three to seven mornings. Increase more slowly if headaches become a problem.

_____ 6. Oxytocin, 10 IU every morning.

_____ 7. Choline, 500 milligrams three times a day.

_____ 8. Inositol, 500 milligrams three times a day.

_____ 9. Triestrogen (natural estrogen), 2.5 milligrams, _____ capsules once a day.

_____ 10. Progesterone (natural), 200 milligrams once a day for the first fourteen days of every month or _____ milligrams once a day.

_____ 11. Testosterone, _____ milligrams, one shot every _____ weeks; or _____ milligrams once a day.

ANTIFUNGALS

_____ 1. Acidophilus or other milk bacteria, 4 billion IU once a day. Take with milk, if you can. Make sure that the brand you buy needs to be refrigerated.

_____ 2. Nystatin, 500,000 IU, two tablets four times a day for approximately five to eight months. Begin with one tablet a day and increase by one tablet a day. If symptoms flare, increase the dose more slowly or stop the medication completely until the symptoms decrease.

_____ 3. Diflucan or Sporanox, 200 milligrams once a
            day for six weeks. Take with food. *Do not take if
            you are using Seldane, Hismanal, or Propulcid.*
            Begin four weeks after starting nystatin.
            If symptoms flared with the nystatin, begin
            with 50 to 100 milligrams a day for one week.
            If symptoms improve but then worsen when
            course is completed, continue the medication
            for another six weeks. *Note: A six-week supply
            costs more than $500.*

ANTIPARASITICS

_____ 1. Flagyl, _____ milligrams three times a day for
            _____ days. Do not drink alcohol while on this
            medication, as this can cause vomiting.
_____ 2. Yodoxin, 650 milligrams three times a day for
            twenty days.
_____ 3. *Artemisia annua,* 500 milligrams, two tablets
            three times a day for twenty days.
_____ 4. Tricyclin, two tablets three times a day for six
            to eight weeks. Take after meals.

NONSPECIFIC TREATMENTS

_____ 1. Nitroglycerin, one-quarter to one tablet
            dissolved under the tongue as needed.
_____ 2. *Rhus toxicodendron* (homeopathic treatment),
            dissolved under the tongue as directed on the
            bottle.
_____ 3. Naphazoline hydrochloride, 1-percent solution,
            one drop in each eye four times a day as
            needed.
_____ 4. Nimodipine, 30 milligrams _____ times a day.
_____ 5. Mexiletine, 150 milligrams _____ times a day.
_____ 6. Pyridostigmine, 30 milligrams _____ times a day.
_____ 7. Hydralazine, 10 to 25 milligrams _____ times
            a day.
_____ 8. Zantac, 150 milligrams twice a day.

_____ 9. Zoloft, _____ milligrams, _____ tablets every morning or evening.

_____ 10. Paxil, 20 milligrams, _____ tablets every morning.

_____ 11. Prozac, 20 milligrams, _____ tablets every morning.

_____ 12. Effexor, 37.5 to 75 milligrams twice a day.

_____ 13. Serzone, 150 milligrams twice a day. Begin with 100 milligrams twice a day for one week.

_____ 14. Neurontin (gabapentin), _____ milligrams _____ times a day.

Information on Commonly Used Treatments for Chronic Fatigue Syndrome and Fibromyalgia

Nutritional Treatments

- *TwinLab Daily One Caps.* This is an excellent multivitamin containing good levels of the B vitamins as well as other vitamins and minerals. Take one each morning. It will turn your urine bright yellow. If it upsets your stomach, take it with food and/or at bedtime, or switch to Centrum multivitamins, one each morning. If you tolerate the Centrum satisfactorally, try adding a B-complex vitamin, one-half of a 50-milligram tablet, at a separate time of day. If your stomach continues to be upset, tell your doctor. Taking a good multivitamin is critical.

- *Magnesium chloride and lactate.* Magnesium is a mineral that is critical for helping tight muscles relax and for treating fatigue. The average American takes in only 250 to 275 milligrams of magnesium through the diet each day because of food processing. A normal diet, such as an Asian diet, supplies approximately 650 milligrams a day. Magnesium is involved in over eighty different reactions in the body and is a critical supplement for treating CFS and fibromyalgia. Since magnesium oxide tablets are poorly absorbed, we often recommend magnesium chloride or lactate instead. It will take about eight months to replace magnesium deficits. After the eight months, you can decrease your dosage from six to two tablets a day.

Magnesium causes diarrhea in many people. If diarrhea becomes a problem for you, take as much as your stomach comfortably allows. Start with one or two tablets a day and work your way up.

- *Fibrocare and Supermalic.* These are mixtures of magnesium and malic acid. Both are available by mail order. Malic acid is a food supplement that is found in citrus fruits. Studies have found that it helps energy metabolism in muscles and helps against fibromyalgia. We prefer using Fibrocare.

- *L-carnitine.* This is an amino acid (protein). It is available both over-the-counter and by prescription. Since it is very expensive, we prefer writing a prescription for it to make insurance reimbursement easier. Several studies have shown that people with CFS have very low muscle carnitine levels and that their fatigue often decreases and their energy improves after about six weeks of carnitine treatment. If your energy improves, continue taking the lowest dose that maintains the improvement. If you notice no change after six weeks, discontinue the carnitine.

- *Coenzyme Q_{10}.* This is another food supplement that is used by the muscles for energy. It is available at health food stores. It is somewhat expensive, however, and we therefore recommend that you purchase it wholesale by mail order. Some experts feel that the oil-based tablets are absorbed better.

- *Iron.* "Normal" levels for iron are adequate for preventing anemia but not the other signs of iron deficiency, including fatigue. We recommend several brands of iron. Ferrous-Sequels has a stool softener that decreases the tendency toward constipation. Most people also tolerate Chromagen fairly well. Chromagen has the added benefit of being a prescription medication, which means that it is often covered by insurance. Vitron C comes in a lower dose, but it is also easier on the stomach. Iron will often cause constipation and turn the stool black. This is normal. It is important not to take any supplemental iron, except the 10 milligrams in the TwinLab Daily One Caps, within six hours of any thyroid or other hormonal supplement or the hormone will not be absorbed.

- *Vitamin B_{12}.* This is a very important vitamin in CFS and fibromyalgia. The current "normal" levels are adequate for preventing anemia, but numerous studies have shown that deficiencies from levels that are well within what is traditionally considered the normal range have caused severe neurologic and psychologic dysfunction. Because of this, we recommend treatment with B_{12} shots any time the B_{12} level is less than 540 picograms per milliliter. Although oral B_{12} supplements in high doses—that is, 1,000 micrograms a day—will slowly raise the B_{12} level, they can take years to succeed. A series of B_{12} shots at the beginning of treatment will raise the level faster. When their course of shots is completed, most patients find that their multivitamins adequately maintain their B_{12} levels.

Sleeping Aids for Fibromyalgia

Do not drive while you are sedated by any medicine.

When taking a sedative, begin with a low dose—approximately one-eighth to one tablet—and work your way up to a dose that helps you sleep through the night without sedating you too much the next day. Initially, take the medication in early evening—for example, around 7:00—so that it has a chance to wear off earlier the next day. Next-day sedation usually disappears in two to three weeks. If you cannot tolerate the medication that your doctor has prescribed, call your doctor to arrange to try another medication.

- *Elavil (amitriptyline).* At doses of up to 300 milligrams per day, Elavil is used as an antidepressant and for nerve injury. We use it for fibromyalgia because it increases the deeper states of sleep that patients are missing. We also use a dose that is tiny in comparison to those used for other illnesses. The medication is not addictive. It is often very sedating, however. Sedation can be decreased by starting with a very low dose, about 5 to 10 milligrams, and slowly working up to one that helps you get a solid night's sleep without being too hung over the next day. The main side effects include dry mouth, constipation, mild weight gain, and, rarely, difficulty urinating. Do not use more than 100 milligrams per night without first checking with your doctor.

- *Flexeril (cyclobenzaprine).* This is a muscle relaxant. The usual dose is one tablet three times a day. We use it primarily to help normalize the sleep cycle. The dose for sleep is one-half to two tablets at bedtime. The main side effects are sedation, dry mouth, and mild weight gain.

- *Desyrel (trazodone)*. This is usually used, at doses of 300 milligrams a day, as a calming agent. It is not addictive and it is sedating. Rarely, males can have prolonged erections—that is, erections that last for more than an hour. If this occurs, call your doctor immediately.

- *Ambien (zolpidem)*. This is a sleeping pill. The usual dose is 5 to 20 milligrams at bedtime. It does not worsen the sleep cycle the way other sleeping pills do, and it does not seem to be addictive, even though the Food and Drug Administration (FDA) requires that this be listed as a side effect. Ambien causes fewer side effects than do most of the other sleep medications listed above.

- *Herbal remedies*. These can be very helpful and nonaddictive. They include valerian root, passionflower, lemon balm, hops, and camomile. They are generally considered to be very safe. They are all available by mail order.

- *Melatonin*. This is a naturally occurring hormone that helps regulate the day-night cycle. It is available in health food stores. It should be taken only in the evening. The usual dose is .3 milligram (one-tenth of a 3-milligram capsule).

- *Klonopin (clonazepam)*. This is a very powerful muscle relaxant. Since it is mildly addictive, we reserve it for our more severe cases. It is very sedating and needs to be started at a very low dose—for example, one-quarter to one tablet at bedtime. It can be increased by one-half to one tablet every three days until a total dose of four tablets (2 milligrams) a day is reached. Do not exceed this dose without first consulting your doctor. For severe muscle spasm, this medication can be taken three to four times a day. If sleep is a major problem, take it mainly at bedtime.

- *Soma (carisoprodol)*. This muscle relaxant is usually taken three to four times a day to treat muscle spasm. One tablet at night can help sleep.

Hormonal Treatments

- *Synthroid.* This is T_4, the main form that thyroid hormone takes in the body. Many people have an underactive thyroid despite technically normal blood tests and often get dramatic relief from treating a subclinical deficiency. The dosing that we use is usually very low and generally will not cause any side effects. Rarely, caffeinelike side effects—for example, shakiness or palpitations—are experienced if the dose is a little too high. If these occur, reduce the dose and also take 200 milligrams of vitamin B_1 daily. If underlying angina is a problem, this medication can unmask it. If you experience chest pain, discontinue the medication and call your doctor immediately. This happens very rarely; we have never seen it with the low dosing that we use. Take Synthroid in the morning.

- *Armour Thyroid.* This is natural thyroid, and it contains a mixture of the body's two most common thyroid hormones, T_3 and T_4. It is best taken in the morning. The side effects are the same as those of Synthroid. Despite this, patients who do not improve with one form of thyroid often dramatically improve with the other.

- *Cortef.* This is cortisol, an adrenal hormone. When cortisol is low, people often feel fatigued, are unable to deal with stress, and have recurrent infections that take a long time to resolve. Low cortisol is also associated with hypoglycemic symptoms and lightheadedness. The dose that we use is very low and usually not associated with side effects, except an occasional acid stomach. Higher doses can cause unmasking of a tendency toward high blood pressure or diabetes, as well as osteoporosis or other severe side effects. These side effects are generally not seen with doses under 35 milligrams a day. We usually know if treatment will be successful within two to three weeks. During periods of physical stress, such as illness, you should double your dose for four to five days. If you become ill, need to undergo any surgery, or have another major problem, notify your doctor immediately.

- *DHEA.* This is another adrenal hormone that is often low in CFS patients. It is the hormone that the adrenal gland produces in the greatest amount. Scientists are just discovering DHEA's functions in the human body. DHEA normally decreases with age. Low DHEA levels are associated with increased risk of heart disease, diabetes, and possibly cancer. Higher levels are associated with longer life and a sense of well-being. Research has shown that if their levels are low, people often feel fatigued. CFS patients often feel much better when they are treated for low DHEA. Side effects are rare. They include acne and increased hair growth on the extremities and, rarely, on the face. It is important to monitor the blood levels to make sure that they stay within the optimum range. We usually know if treatment will be successful within two to three weeks. DHEA can be obtained only by mail order from compounding pharmacies.

- *Florinef.* This is a hormone that helps to conserve salt and water. Many CFS patients have increased thirst and a tendency toward low blood pressure and dizziness. Recent research has shown that many CFS symptoms improve with Florinef treatment. It can take up to three months to see the full benefit. Start slowly with one-quarter of a .1-milligram tablet every morning. Increase to one-half tablet daily the second week, three-quarters tablet daily the third week, and then a whole tablet daily the fourth week. Get plenty of salt and water, as well as extra potassium from sources such as bananas and Campbell's V-8 Juice.

- *Oxytocin.* This is a hypothalamic hormone and neurotransmitter. It is most often thought of as the hormone that induces labor. Although we are just learning what its role is in other body functions, some researchers have found that patients feel better when they are treated for low levels. If treatment will help, improvement is usually evident within two weeks. The dose that we use is the dose that the body reportedly puts out during orgasm. There is no blood test to check the level in the body, so treatment is started if symptoms that suggest deficiency are present. These symptoms include cold hands, cold feet, pallor, and decreased short-term memory, as well as other symptoms commonly seen in CFS and fibromyalgia. Oxytocin is available by mail order.

- *Choline and inositol.* Taking 500 milligrams three times a day of each can make oxytocin treatment more effective. Begin the choline and inositol six weeks before the oxytocin. Side effects are rare.

Antifungals

- *Acidophilus and other milk bacteria.* Take 3 to 6 billion IU daily. These friendly bacteria compete with the yeast. To help them do their job, avoid sugar and other sweeteners, which help yeast to grow, and add fructooligosaccharides (FOS).

- *Nystatin.* This is a very benign antifungal. In itself, it rarely causes side effects, except occasional mild nausea, because at the doses we recommend, it is not absorbed into the body. Rather, it stays in the bowel and is excreted. However, when a person has a yeast problem and the yeast is rapidly killed off, the yeast symptoms tend to flare. Because of this, we recommend beginning the treatment slowly, increasing the daily dose by one tablet every one to four days until the recommended dose is reached. If symptoms do flare, reduce the dose again until the symptoms subside and then slowly begin increasing the dose once more. We usually recommend continuing nystatin for about five to eight months to help clear any yeast overgrowth in the bowel. Unfortunately, the concept of yeast overgrowth is very controversial and there are no definitive tests to define the difference between normal yeast growth and overgrowth. We can see skin conditions such as athlete's foot and thrush. When the overgrowth is inside the body, however, we must treat based on suspicion. This is why we recommend taking a stool test and filling out the yeast questionnaire.

- *Diflucan and Sporanox.* These are very powerful yet safe antifungals. Unfortunately, they are also very expensive. Most of the studies undertaken in the United States using these treatments were done on patients with acquired immune deficiency syndrome (AIDS). These patients suffer horrible side effects from most medications, even common sulfa antibiotics. In European studies done on patients with moderate yeast overgrowth but not AIDS, the side-effect profile was good. Diflucan and Sporanox were repeatedly shown to be very safe agents. Once in a rare while, liver inflammation occurs. However, we have not seen this with Sporanox. *Do not use either Diflucan or Sporanox if you are taking the antihistamine Seldane or Hismanal or the bowel medicine Propulcid.* In addition, Sporanox must be taken with food or absorption is reduced by 40 percent. If the recommended dosage is two tablets or capsules a day, they should be taken together. Diflucan or Sporanox should also be taken in conjunction with nystatin. We usually recommend a six-week course. If symptoms improve but then recur when the medication is stopped, repeat the six-week course.

Antiparasitics

- *Flagyl (metronidazole).* This is a common antiparasitic agent. Its main side effect is nausea, which is not dangerous but can be a nuisance. Drinking alcohol causes vomiting. You may feel worse for one to three weeks while the parasites die off.

- *Yodoxin.* This is an antiamoebic. The main side effect is mild nausea.

- *Artemisia annua and tricyclin.* These are herbal antiparasitic remedies. The main, though uncommon, side effect is nausea. We recommend taking two 500-milligram artemisia capsules three times a day for twenty days. For tricyclin, our recommendation is two tablets three times a day, after meals, for six to eight weeks.

Nonspecific Treatments

- *Nitroglycerin, nimodipine, mexiletine, hydralazine, Zantac, etc.* These medications generally are used for other medical problems but have been found to be helpful against fibromyalgia or CFS. As they are not used that often, your doctor will discuss them with you if and when he or she prescribes them.

- *Zoloft, Paxil, Prozac, Effexor, and Serzone.* These are nonaddictive antidepressant agents. They tend to increase the body's levels of serotonin, which is a neurotransmitter. They are usually not sedating but often have an energizing effect, even in the absence of depression. Because of this, they can be useful against fatigue in patients who are not clinically depressed. Also because of this, they should be taken in the morning to allow the effect to wear off by evening. Patients who are sedated by these medications, however, should take them at night. Some patients experience delayed orgasm when taking these agents. This side effect is least likely with Serzone.

If you become too shaky when taking one of these medications, start slowly—one-quarter to one-half tablet the first week, increasing by one-quarter to one-half tablet every week until the desired dose is reached. The maximum dose for all these medications is usually two to four tablets daily. If you need to take more than two tablets at one time, take two in the morning and two at lunchtime. Do not increase the dose beyond what your doctor recommended without first getting the doctor's approval. It takes six weeks to see the full effect of any of these agents.

Appendix G

Patient Support Groups

NATIONAL GROUPS

American Association for
  Chronic Fatigue Syndrome
P.O. Box 895
Olney, Maryland 20830
*An umbrella organization focusing
on scientific research.*

Arthritis Foundation
P.O. Box 19000
Atlanta, Georgia 30326
(800) 283–7800

Candida Research Foundation
1638 B Street
Hayward, California 94541
(510) 582–2179

CFIDS Activation Network
  (CAN)
P.O. Box 345
Larchmont, New York 10538
(914) 627–5631

Chronic Fatigue and Immune
  Dsyfunction Syndrome
  Association of America

P.O. Box 220398
Charlotte, North Carolina
  28222-0398
(800) 442–3437
*An excellent national patient
support group and educational
resource.*

Chronic Fatigue and Immune
  Dysfunction Syndrome
  Pathfinder
P.O. Box 2644
Kensington, Maryland
  20891-2644
(301) 530–8624

Chronic Fatigue Syndrome
  Crisis Center
27 West 20th Street
Suite 703
New York, New York 10011
(212) 691–4800
(212) 691–5113 (FAX)

Chronic Fatigue Syndrome
  Foundation
10 Wild Partridge Court

Greensboro, North Carolina
  27455
(919) 288-2893
(800) 597-4237

Chronic Fatigue Syndrome/
  Myalgic Encephalitis
  Computer Networking Project
P.O. Box 11347
Washington, D.C. 20008
cfs-me@sjuvm,stjohns.edu
  (email)

Chronicles of Chronic Fatigue
  and Immune Dysfunction
  Syndrome
John Friedrich
P.O. Box 465
Ashland, Massachusetts 01721

Compuserve Chronic Fatigue
  and Immune Dysfunction
  Syndrome Support Area
CFS/CFIDS/FMS Section (16)
Health and Fitness Forum
  (Good Health)
(505) 898-4635
  (CFIDS information)
(800) 898-8199
  (Compuserve information)

Fibromyalgia Network
5700 Stockdale Highway #100
Bakersfield, California 93309
(805) 631-1950
*This is a "must join" group for
fibromyalgia patients.*

Food Allergy Network
747 Holly Avenue
Fairfax, Virginia 22030-5647
(800) 929-4040

Myalgic Encephalitis Association
  of Canada
246 Queen Street

Suite 400
Ottawa, Ontario K1P 5E4
Canada
(613) 563-1565
*An excellent source of general
information for CFIDS and
fibromyalgia patients, as well as
a good source of important
information for Canadian patients.*

National Chronic Fatigue
  Syndrome and Fibromyalgia
  Association
P.O. Box 18426
Kansas City, Missouri 64133
(816) 931-4777

National Myalgic Encephalitis/
  Fibromyalgia Action Network
3836 Carling Avenue
Highway 17B
Nepean, Ontario K2H 7V2
Canada
(613) 829-6667

National Organization for
  Seasonal Affective Disorder
P.O. Box 40133
Washington, D.C. 20016

Nightingale Research
  Foundation
383 Danforth Avenue
Ottawa, Ontario K2A OE3
Canada

Well Spouse Foundation
P.O. Box 801
New York, New York 10023
(212) 724-7209

LOCAL AND REGIONAL GROUPS

Chicago Chronic Fatigue
  Syndrome Association
818 Wenonah Avenue

Oak Park, Illinois 60304
(708) 524–9322

Chronic Fatigue and Immune
  Dysfunction Syndrome Society
South Coast Chapter
Linda Coffey, Group Leader
5200 Heil Avenue #23
Huntington Beach, California
  92647

Chronic Fatigue Syndrome
  Association of Virginia, Inc.
P.O. Box 2337
Glen Allen, Virginia 23058-2337
(804) 330–7518

Connecticut Chronic Fatigue
  and Immune Dysfunction
  Syndrome Association
P.O. Box 9582
Forestville, Connecticut 06011
(203) 582–CFIDS (582–3437)

Essex County Fibromyalgia
  Group
977 University Avenue West
Second Floor
Windsor, Ontario N9A 5S3
Canada
(519) 254–0417

Fibromyalgia Association
  of British Columbia
Box 15455
Vancouver, British Columbia
  V6B 5B2
Canada
(604) 540–0488

Fibromyalgia Association
  of Central Ohio
Riverside Hospital
Suite 8
3545 Olentangy River Road

Columbus, Ohio 43214
(614) 262–2000

Fibromyalgia Association
  of Florida, Inc.
P.O. Box 14848
Gainesville, Florida 32604-4848
(904) 373–6865

Fibromyalgia Association
  of Greater Washington
P.O. Box 2373
Centreville, Virginia 22020
(703) 790–2324

Fibromyalgia Association
  of Northern Virginia
(703) 912–1727

Fibromyalgia Association
  of Texas, Inc.
5650 Forest Lane
Dallas, Texas 75230
(214) 363–2473

Greater New York Chronic
  Fatigue Syndrome Coalition
880 Pine Avenue
West Islip, New York 11795
(516) 548–8237

Gulf Coast Chronic Fatigue
  Syndrome/Chronic Fatigue
  and Immune Dysfunction
  Syndrome Association
752 J Avenue Estancias
Venice, Florida 34292-2316
(813) 484–0706

Los Angeles Chronic Fatigue
  and Immune Dysfunction
  Syndrome Association
P.O. Box 5414
Sherman Oaks, California 91413
(818) 785–8301
(818) 458–9092 (recorded
  information line)

Massachusetts Chronic Fatigue
and Immune Dysfunction
Syndrome Association
808 Main Street
Waltham, Massachusetts 02154
(617) 893-4415

Ontario Fibrositis Association
250 Bloor Street East #401
Toronto M4W 3P2
Canada
(416) 967-1414

Rhode Island Chronic Fatigue
and Immune Dysfunction
Syndrome Association
UPC Building
500 Prospect Street
Pawtucket, Rhode Island 02860
(401) 729-0019

San Francisco Chronic Fatigue
and Immune Dysfunction
Syndrome Foundation
965 Mission Street
Suite 425
San Francisco, California 94103
(415) 882-9986

Southern California Chronic
Fatigue and Immune
Dysfunction Syndrome
Support Network

23732 Hillhurst Drive #U-9
Laguna Niguel, California 92677
(714) 249-6976

Utah Chronic Fatigue and
Immune Dysfunction
Syndrome Association, Inc.
P.O. Box 511257
Salt Lake City, Utah 84151
(801) 461-3378

Wisconsin Chronic Fatigue
Syndrome Association
P.O. Box 442
Thiensville, Wisconsin 53092
(414) 768-7560

HOTLINES

Chronic Fatigue Syndrome
Hotline
(800) Help-CFS (435-7237)

National Chronic Fatigue
Syndrome and Fibromyalgia
Association Hotline
Kansas City, Missouri
(816) 313-2000

National Chronic Fatigue
Syndrome Hotline
Charleston, South Carolina
(800) 237-2407

Appendix H

Physicians Specializing in Chronic Fatigue Syndrome

Physician Organizations

American College for
  Advancement of Medicine
P.O. Box 3427
Laguna Hills, California 92654
(800) 532-3688
(714) 583-7666

American Holistic Medical
  Association (AHMA)
4101 Lake Boone Trail
Suite 201
Raleigh, North Carolina 27607
(919) 787-5146
*Provides speakers through its
Speakers Bureau.*

Physicians

ALABAMA

Robert E. Pieroni, M.D.
Professor of Internal Medicine
University of Alabama
Tuscaloosa, Alabama 35487
(205) 348-1287

CALIFORNIA

Jay Goldstein, M.D.
6200 East Canyon Rim Road
  #110D
Anaheim Hills, California 92807
(714) 998-2780

Michael Rosenbaum, M.D.
45 San Clemente Drive
Suite B-130
Corte Madera, California 94925
(415) 927-9450

Murray Susser, M.D.
2730 Wilshire Boulevard
Suite 110
Santa Monica, California 90403
(310) 453-4424
*Coauthored "Solving the Puzzle of
Chronic Fatigue Syndrome."*

Julian Whitaker, M.D.
Wellness Institute
4321 Birth Street
Suite 100
Newport Beach, California
  92660
(714) 851-1550

DISTRICT OF COLUMBIA

Alexander Chester, M.D.
3301 New Mexico Avenue, NW
Suite 348
Washington, D.C. 20016
(202) 362-4467
*Specializes in nasal congestion
and CFS.*

George Mitchell, M.D.
2639 Connecticut Avenue, NW
  #C-100
Washington, D.C. 20008
(202) 265-4092
*Specializes in clinical ecology and
environmental sensitivity.*

ILLINOIS

Chronic Fatigue Syndrome
  Center
Sigita Plioplys, M.D.
Audrius Plioplys, M.D.
Mercy Hospital
Chicago, Illinois 60616
(312) 445-0123
Carnitine researchers.

MARYLAND

James Brodsky, M.D.
4701 Willand Avenue #224
Chevy Chase, Maryland
  20815
(301) 652-6760

Robert Greenfield, M.D.
Alan Weiss, M.D.
139 Old Solomons Island Road
Annapolis, Maryland 21401
(410) 224-2222

Richard Layton, M.D.
901 Dulaney Valley Road

Towson, Maryland
  21204
(410) 337-2707
*Specializes in clinical ecology
and allergies.*

Norman Rosen, M.D.
8415 Bellona Lane
Towson, Maryland 21404
(410) 821-7775
Specializes in physiatry.

Jacob Teitelbaum, M.D.
466 Forelands Road
Annapolis, Maryland 21401
(410) 573-5389

MICHIGAN

Ruth Walkotten, D.O.
427 West Siminole Road
Muskegon, Michigan
  49441
(616) 733-1989

NEW HAMPSHIRE

Rex G. Carr, M.D.
Building 1
Suite 9B
One Oak Ridge Road
West Lebanon, New Hampshire
  03784
(603) 643-5254
*Specializes in physical medicine
and rehabilitation.*

NEW JERSEY

Richard Podell, M.D., M.P.H.
571 Central Avenue
Suite 106
New Providence, New Jersey
  07974
(908) 464-3800

NEW YORK

Leo Galland, M.D.
133 East 73rd Street
New York, New York 10021
(212) 861–9000
Specializes in parasitic infections.

NORTH CAROLINA

Paul Cheney, M.D., Ph.D
10620 Park Road #234
Charlotte, North Carolina 28210

Jorge D. Flechas, M.D.
724 5th Avenue West
Hendersonville, North Carolina
    28739
(704) 693–3015
Uses DHEA and oxytocin.

Charles Lapp, M.D.
10724 Park Road

Suite 105
Building 100
Mercy South Medical Park
Charlotte, North Carolina 28210
(704) 543–9692

TEXAS

Thomas Steinbach, M.D.
902 Frostwood #243
Houston, Texas 77024
(713) 467–6471
Specializes in kutapressin research.

CANADA

Byron Hyde, M.D.
Nightingale Research
    Foundation
Ottawa, Ontario K2A 0E3
Canada

Appendix I

Mail Order Sources

MEDICATIONS, SUPPLEMENTS, AND HERBAL REMEDIES

Allergy Research
400 Preda Street
San Leandro, California 94577
(800) 782-4274
*Sells tricyclin, an antiparasitic
herbal preparation. A prescription
is necessary.*

Belmar Pharmacy
12860 West Cedar Drive
Lakewood, Colorado 80228
(800) 525-9473
*Carries DHEA and oxytocin
tablets. The physician phones in
the prescription as well as the
patient's credit card number,
and Belmar mails the medication
directly to the patient.*

Cape Apothecary
1384 Cape Saint Claire Road
Annapolis, Maryland 21401
(410) 974-1788
(800) 248-5978
*Good source for triestrogen and
natural progesterone.*

CFIDS Buyers Club
1187 Coast Village Road

#1-280
Santa Barbara, California 93108
(800) 366-6056
*Carries many of the nonprescrip-
tion supplements that CFS patients
need, including oil-based coenzyme
Q10 tablets. Most of the prices are
very competitive, and some of the
profits go to CFIDS research.
I strongly recommend this group.*

Ecologic Formulas
1061-B Shary Circle
Concord, California 94518
(800) 888-4585
*Sells 150 Tonic Mineral Formula
I, a magnesium-potassium
aspartate product.*

Herb Finders
P.O. Box 3868
Salt Lake City, Utah
    84110-3868
(800) 780-6934
Carries turkey rhubarb.

Metagenics
166 Fernwood Avenue
Adison, New Jersey 08837
(800) 638-2848
or

Steven Nadell, Representative
4403 Vineland Road B-10
Orlando, Florida 32811
(800) 647-6100
*Sells Ultraclear, a hypoallergenic
powdered food to use with
elimination diets. Also ask for
the instruction booklet.*

Optimox
P.O. Box 3378
Torrance, California 90510
(800) 223-1601
*Carries magnesium with malic
acid, as well as general vitamins.*

To Your Health
11809 Nightingale Circle
Fountain Hills, Arizona 85268
(800) 801-1406
*Carries Fibrocare, as well as
Valerian Rest, a valerian root–
lemon balm herbal remedy
for sleep. Also has an excellent
resource and supply catalogue for
fibromyalgia and CFIDS.*

Vitamin Shoppe
4700 West Side Avenue
North Bergen, New Jersey 07047
(201) 866-7711
(800) 223-1216
*Its Zinc Lozenges Plus are excellent
against respiratory infections.
Also carries magnesium-potassium
aspartate and Super Snooze.*

PRODUCTS

Bearhard Industries
300 71st Street
Suite 435
Miami Beach, Florida 33141
(305) 861-2536
*Sells a nasal steamer that is
excellent for sinus problems.*

Bio Brite
7315 Wisconsin Avenue
Suite 1300 West
Bethesda, Maryland 20814
(301) 961-8557
(800) 621-LITE (621-5483)
*Sells light boxes and light visors
for persons suffering from seasonal
affective disorder.*

CNS
4400 West 78st Street
Bloomington, Minnesota 55435
(612) 820-6696
*Distributor of Breathe Right Nasal
Strips.*

Pure Water
Bren Jacobson
103 Second Street
Annapolis, Maryland 21401
(410) 224-4877
*Consultant on health and environ-
mental concerns, especially water,
and distributor of several brands of
water filters, including Multipure.*

BODY WORK AND COUNSELING/INNER WORK

**Association for Transpersonal
   Psychology**
P.O. Box 3049
Stanford, California 94309
(415) 327-2066
(415) 327-0535 (FAX)
http://www.igc.org/atp/
   (World Wide Web site)
For referrals to wholistic counselors.

Brugh Joy, Inc.
P.O. Box 670
Paulden, Arizona 86334
(800) 448-9187
For information on workshops.

The Guild for
Structural Integration
P.O. Box 1559
Boulder, Colorado 80306
(800) 447-0150
For practitioners of the Rolf method
of structural integration.

Restless Leg Foundation
P.O. Box 314-JH
514 Daniels Street
Raleigh, North Carolina 27605
For information on restless leg
syndrome.

Rolf Institute
205 Canyon Boulevard
Boulder, Colorado 80302
(303) 449-5903
(800) 530-8875
For information and referrals.

Trager Institute
21 Locust Avenue
Mill Valley, California 94941
(415) 388-2688

(415) 388-2710 (FAX)
TragerD@trager.com (email)
For referrals to instructors, tutors,
and practitioners.

LAB TESTING

Great Smoky Mountain Lab
18A Regent Park Boulevard
Asheville, North Carolina 28806
(800) 522-4762
Does an excellent job with stool
testing.

Jacob Teitelbaum, M.D.
466 Forelands Road
Annapolis, Maryland 21401
(410) 573-5389
(800) 333-5287
For information on and test kits
for blood and stool testing. Also
offers interpretations of blood
tests processed in other labs and
treatment recommendations based
on lab testing.

Notes

INTRODUCTION

1. J. Teitelbaum and B. Bird, "Effective Treatment of Severe Chronic Fatigue: A Report of a Series of 64 Patients," *Journal of Musculoskeletal Pain* 3 (1995): 91–110.

CHAPTER 1

1. G. P. Holmes, J. E. Kaplan, et al., "Chronic Fatigue Syndrome: A Working Case Definition," *Annals of Internal Medicine* 108 (1988): 387–389.
2. R. K. Price, C. S. North, et al., "Estimating the Presence of Chronic Fatigue Syndrome in the Community," *Public Health Reports* 107 (September–October 1992): 514–522.
3. R. B. Marchesani, "Critical Antiviral Pathway Deficient in Chronic Fatigue Syndrome Patients," *Infectious Disease News*, August 1993, p. 4.
4. D. L. Goldenberg, "Fibromyalgia Syndrome," *Journal of the American Medical Association* 257 (1987): 2782–2787.
5. S. E. Strauss, S. Fritz, J. K. Dale, B. Gould, and W. Strober, "Lymphocyte Phenotype and Function in Chronic Fatigue Syndrome," *Journal of Clinical Immunology* 13 (January 1993): 30–40.
6. J. Teitelbaum and B. Bird, "Effective Treatment of Severe Chronic Fatigue: A Report of a Series of 64 Patients," *Journal of Musculoskeletal Pain* 3 (1995): 91–110.
7. D. Halpin and S. Wessely, "VP-1 Antigen in Chronic Postviral Fatigue Syndrome," *Lancet*, 1989, pp. 1028–1029.
8. G. E. Yousef, E. J. Bell, et al., "Chronic Enterovirus Infection in Patients With Postviral Fatigue Syndrome," *Lancet*, 1988, pp. 146–147.
9. L. E. Archard, N. E. Bowles, P. O. Behan, et al., "Postviral Fatigue Syndrome Persistence of Enterovirus RNA in Muscle and Elevated Creatine Kinase,"

Journal of the Royal Society of Medicine 81 (1988): 326–329.

10. D. Wakefield, A. Lloyd, and J. Dwyer, "Human Herpes Virus 6 and Myalgic Encephalomyelitis," *Lancet*, 1988, p. 1059.

11. W. Jeffries, *Safe Uses of Cortisone*, monograph (Springfield, IL: Charles C. Thomas, 1981).

12. B. M. Hyde, ed., *The Clinical and Scientific Basis of Myalgic Encephalitis and Chronic Fatigue Syndrome* (Ottawa, ON: Nightingale Research Foundation, 1992).

13. G. Neeck and W. Riedel, "Thyroid Function in Patients With Fibromyalgia Syndrome," *Journal of Rheumatology* 19 (1992): 1120–1122.

14. M. A. Demitrack, J. K. Dale, S. E. Strauss, L. Lave, S. J. Listwak, and M. J. Kreuss, "Evidence for Impaired Activation of the Hypothalamic-Pituitary-Adrenal Axis in Patients With Chronic Fatigue Syndrome," *Journal of Clinical Endocrinology and Metabolism* 73 (1991): 1223–1234.

15. G. A. McCain and K. S. Tilbe, "Diurnal Hormone Variation in Fibromyalgia Syndrome and a Comparison With Rheumatoid Arthritis," *Journal of Rheumatology* 25 (1993): 469–474.

16. A.M.O. Bakheit, P. O. Behan, T. G. Dinan, et al., "Possible Upregulation of Hypothalamic 5-HT Receptors in Patients With Postviral Fatigue Syndrome," *Boston Medical Journal* 304 (April 1992): 1010–1012.

17. E. N. Griep, J. N. Boersma, et al., "Altered Reactivity of the HPA Axis in the Primary Fibromyalgia Syndrome," *Journal of Rheumatology* 20 (1993): 469–474.

CHAPTER 2

1. R. M. Marston and B. B. Peterkin, "Nutrient Content of the National Food Supply," *National Food Review*, Winter 1980, pp. 21–25.

2. J. H. Nelson, "Wheat—Its Processing and Utilization," *American Journal of Clinical Nutrition* 41, supplement (May 1985): 1070–1076.

3. H. A. Schroeder, "Loss of Vitamins and Trace Minerals Resulting From Processing and Preservation of Foods," *American Journal of Clinical Nutrition* 24 (May 1971): 562–573.

4. S. B. Eaton, "Paleolithic Nutrition," *New England Journal of Medicine* 312 (31 January 1985): 283–289.

5. H. C. Trowell, ed., *Western Diseases: Their Emergence and Prevention* (Cambridge, MA: Harvard University Press, 1981).

6. W. Mertz, ed., "Beltsville 1 Year Dietary Intake Survey," *American Journal of Clinical Nutrition* 40, supplement (December 1984): 1323–1403.

7. W. G. Crook, *The Yeast Connection and the Woman* (Jackson, TN: Professional Books, 1995).

8. J. G. Travell and D. G. Simons, *Myofascial Pain and Dysfunction: The Trigger Point Manual*, vol. 1 (Baltimore, MD: Williams & Wilkins, 1983), pp. 103–164.

9. B. Kennes, et al., "Effect of Vitamin C Supplements on Cell-Mediated Immunity in Old People," *Gerontology* 29 (1983): 305–310.

10. R. K. Chandra, "Effect of Macro and Micro Nutrient Deficiencies and Excess on Immune Response," *Food Technology*, February 1985, pp. 91–93.

11. S. Chandra, et al., "Undernutrition Impairs Immunity," *Internal Medicine* 5 (December 1984): 85–99.

12. R. K. Chandra, et al., "NIH Workshop on Trace Element Regulation of Immunity and Infection," *Nutrition Research* 2 (1982): 721–733.

13. M. C. Talbott, "Pyridoxine Supplementation: Effect on Lymphocyte Responses in Elderly Persons," *American Journal of Clinical Nutrition* 46 (1987): 659–664.

14. S. N. Meydani, et al., "Vitamin E Supplementation Enhances Cell-Mediated Immunity in Healthy Elderly Subjects," *American Journal of Clinical Nutrition* 52 (1990): 557–563.

15. E. Braunwald, ed., *Harrisons Principles of Internal Medicine*, 11th ed. (New York: McGraw-Hill, 1987), p. 1496.

16. T. Walter, et al., *American Journal of Clinical Nutrition* 44 (1986): 877–882.

17. T. F. Kirn, "Do Low Levels of Iron Affect Body's Ability to Regulate Temperature, Experience Cold?" *Journal of the American Medical Association* 260 (5 August 1988): 607.

18. L. S. Darnell, "Abstract 21," *American Journal of Clinical Nutrition*, supplement.

19. D. C. Rushton, et al., "Letters to the Editor," *Lancet*, 22 June 1991, p. 1554.

20. J. Lindenbaum, E. B. Healton, et al., "Neuropsychiatric Disorders Caused by Cobalamin Deficiency in the Absence of Anemia or Macrocytoses," *New England Journal of Medicine* 318 (1988): 1720–1728.

21. W. S. Beck, "Cobalamin and the Nervous System," *New England Journal of Medicine* 318, editorial (1988): 1752–1754.

22. J. Lindenbaum, et al., "Prevalence of Cobalamin Deficiency in the Framingham Elderly Population," *American Journal of Clinical Nutrition* 60 (1994): 2–11.

23. D. S. Karnaze, et al., "Low Serum Cobalmin Levels in Primary Degenerative Dementia: Do Some Patients Harbor Atypical Cobalmin Deficiency States?" *Archives of Internal Medicine* 147 (1987): 429–431.

24. M. S. Seelig, "The Requirement of Magnesium by the Normal Adult," *American Journal of Clinical Nutrition* 14 (June 1964): 342–390.

25. F. L. Lakshmanad, et al., "Magnesium Intakes and Balances," *American Journal of Clinical Nutrition* 40, supplement (December 1984): 1380–1389.

26. M.J.A.J.M. Hoes, "Plasma Concentrations of Magnesium and Vitamin B₁ in Alcoholism and Delirium Tremans," *Acta*

Psychiatrica Belgica 81 (1981): 72–84.

CHAPTER 3

1. J. Teitelbaum and B. Bird, "Effective Treatment of Severe Chronic Fatigue: A Report of a Series of 64 Patients," *Journal of Musculoskeletal Pain* 3 (1995): 91–110.
2. W. Jeffries, *Safe Uses of Cortisone*, monograph (Springfield, IL: Charles C. Thomas, 1981).
3. W. Jeffries, letter to author, 31 July 1993.
4. R. A. Anderson, et al., "Chromium and Hypoglycemia," *American Journal of Clinical Nutrition* 41, abstract (April 1985): 841.
5. W. Jeffries, "Low Dose Glucocorticoid Therapy," *Archives of Internal Medicine* 119 (1967): 265–278.
6. P.M.J. Zelissen, et al., "Effect of Glucocorticord Replacement Therapy on Bone Mineral Density in Patients With Addison's Disease," *Annals of Internal Medicine* 120 (1994): 207–210.
7. A. W. Meikle, et al., "Adrenal Androgen Secretion and Biologic Effects," *Endocrine and Metabolic Clinics of North America* 20 (June 1991): 381–421.
8. L. N. Parker, "Control of Adrenal Androgen Secretion," *Endocrine and Metabolic Clinics of North America* 20 (June 1991): 401–421.
9. E. Barrett-Connor, R. T. Khaw, and S. C. Yen, "A Prospective Study of DHEA, Mortality and Cardiovascular Disease," *New England Journal of Medicine* 315 (1986): 1519–1524.
10. P. C. Rowe, I. Bole-Hoiaighah, J. S. Kan, and H. Calkins, "Is Neurally Mediated Hypotension an Unrecognized Cause of Chronic Fatigue?" *Lancet* 345 (11 March 1995): 623–624.
11. G. Faglia, et al., "Thyrotropin Secretion in Patients With Central Hypothyroidism," *Journal of Clinical Endocrinology and Metabolism* 48 (1979): 989–998.
12. J. G. Travell and D. G. Simons, *Myofascial Pain and Dysfunction: The Trigger Point Manual*, vol. 1 (Baltimore, MD: Williams & Wilkins, 1983), pp. 103–164.
13. J. Travell, *Archives of Physical Medicine and Rehabilitation* 62 (1981): 100–106.
14. D. G. Simons, "Myofascial Pain Syndrome Due to Trigger Points," *International Rehabilitation Medicine Association Monograph Series* 1 (November 1987).
15. W. Alexander, *Internal Medicine World Report*, 1–14 January 1995, p. 32.
16. R. D. Gambrell, *Consultant*, July 1994, pp. 1047–1057.
17. M. Brock, *Acta Neurochirurgica* 47, supplement (1990): 127–128.
18. J. S. Jenkins, "The Role of Oxytocin: Present Concepts," *Clinical Endocrinology* 34 (1991): 515–525.
19. J. Fletchas, conversation with author, 8 October 1994.
20. M. L. Vance, "Hypopituitarism," *New England Journal of Medicine* 330: 1651–1662.

21. G. A. McGauley, "Quality of Life Assessment Before and After Growth Hormone Treatment in Adults With GH Deficiency," *Acta Paediatrica Scandinavica* 356, supplement (1989): 70–72.

22. R. C. Cuneo, F. Salomen, et al., "GH Treatment in Growth Hormone Deficient Adults," part II: "Effects on Exercise Performance," *Journal of Applied Physiology* 70 (1991): 695–700.

23. J.O.L. Jorgensen, S. A. Pedersen, et al., "Long Term GH Treatment in Growth Hormone Deficient Adults," *Acta Endocrinol (Copenhagen)* 125 (1991): 449–453.

24. R. B. Bennet, S. R. Clark, et al., "Low Levels of Somatomedin C in Patients With the Fibromyalgia Syndrome," *Arthritis and Rheumatism* 35 (1992): 1113–1116.

25. A.M.O. Bakheit, P. O. Behan, et al., "Abnormal Arginine-Vasopressin Secretion and Water Metabolism in Patients With Post-Viral Fatigue Syndrome," *Acta Neurologica Scandinavica* 87 (1993): 234–238.

CHAPTER 4

1. J. R. Quesada, M. Talpaz, et al., "Clinical Toxicity of Interferon in Cancer Patients: A Review," *Journal of Clinical Oncology* 4 (February 1986): 234–243.

2. F. Adams, J. R. Avesada, et al., "Neuropsychiatric Manifestations of Human Leukocyte Interferon Therapy in Patients With Cancer," *Journal of the American Medical Association* 252 (1984): 938–941.

3. A. W. Meikle, et al., "Adrenal Androgen Secretion and Biologic Effects," *Endocrine and Metabolic Clinics of North America* 20 (June 1991): 381–421.

4. E. Barker, S. F. Fujimura, et al., "Immunologic Abnormalities Associated With Chronic Fatigue Syndrome," *Clinical Infectious Diseases* 18, supplement 1 (1994): 5136–5141.

5. T. Aoki, H. Miyakoshi, et al., "Low NK Syndrome and Its Relationship to Chronic Fatigue Syndrome," *Clinical Immunology and Immunopathology* 69 (December 1993): 253–265.

6. W. G. Crook, *The Yeast Connection and the Woman* (Jackson, TN: Professional Books, 1995).

7. G. Reid, "Implantation of Lactobacillus Casei Var Rhamnosus Into Vagina," *Lancet* 344, letter (29 October 1994): 1229.

8. Procter and Gamble Pharmaceuticals, inhouse research data.

9. J. Avorn, "Reduction of Bacteriuria and Pyuria After Ingestion of Cranberry Juice," *Journal of the American Medical Association* 271 (1994): 751–754.

10. J. Edman, et al., "Zinc Status in Women With Recurrent Vulvovaginal Candidiasis," *American Journal of Obstetrics and Gynecology* 155 (1986): 1082–1088.

11. R. Boyne, *Journal of Nutrition* 116 (1982): 816–822.

12. R. J. Deckelbaum, "ELISA More Accurate Than Microscopy for Giardia," *Infectious Diseases in Children*, October 1993, p. 30.

13. G. P. Holmes, J. E. Kaplan, et al., "Chronic Fatigue Syndrome: A Working Case Definition," *Annals of Internal Medicine* 108 (1988): 387–389.

14. L. Galland, et al., "Giardia as a Cause of Chronic Fatigue," *Journal of Nutritional Medicine* 1 (1990): 27–31.

15. A. L. Gittleman, *Guess What Came to Dinner: Parasites and Your Health* (Garden City Park, NY: Avery Publishing Group, 1993).

16. D. G. Simons, "Myofascial Pain Syndrome Due to Trigger Points," *International Rehabilitation Medicine Association Monograph Series* 1 (November 1987).

17. J. G. Travell and D. G. Simons, *Myofascial Pain and Dysfunction: The Trigger Point Manual*, vol. 1 (Baltimore, MD: Williams & Wilkins, 1983), pp. 103–164.

CHAPTER 5

1. J. G. Travell and D. G. Simons, *Myofascial Pain and Dysfunction: The Trigger Point Manual*, vol. 1 (Baltimore, MD: Williams & Wilkins, 1983), pp. 103–164.

2. G. A. McCain and K. S. Tilbe, "Diurnal Hormone Variation in Fibromyalgia Syndrome and a Comparison With Rheumatoid Arthritis," *Journal of Rheumatology* 25 (1993): 469–474.

3. G. Neeck and W. Riedel, "Thyroid Function in Patients With Fibromyalgia Syndrome," *Journal of Rheumatology* 19 (1992): 1120–1122.

4. H. Moldofsky, "Sleep and Chronic Fatigue Syndrome," in *Chronic Fatigue Syndrome*, ed. D. Dawson and S. Sabin (Boston: Little, Brown and Company, 1993).

5. R. M. Bennett, R. A. Gatter, et al., "Cyclobenzaprine Versus Placebo in Fibromyalgia," *Arthritis and Rheumatism* 31 (December 1988): 1535–1542.

6. R. A. Gatter, "Pharmacotherapeutics in Fibromyalgia," *American Journal of Medicine* 81, supplement 3A (29 September 1986): 63–66.

7. H. Dressing and D. Riemann, "Insomnia: Are Valerian/Melissa Combinations of Equal Value to Benzodiazepine?" *Therapiewoche* 42 (1992): 726–736.

CHAPTER 6

1. S. Rogers, *Tired or Toxic* (Syracuse, NY: Prestige Publishing, 1990).

2. S. Rogers, "Chemical Sensitivity: Breaking the Paralyzing Paradigm," part I, *Internal Medicine World Report*, vol. 7, no. 3, p. 1.

3. S. Rogers, "Chemical Sensitivity: Breaking the Paralyzing Paradigm," part II, *Internal Medicine World Report*, vol. 7, no. 6, pp. 8, 21–31.

4. A. C. Chester, "Chronic Fatigue

of Nasal Origin: Possible Confusion With Chronic Fatigue Syndrome," in *The Clinical and Scientific Basis of Myalgic Encephalitis and Chronic Fatigue Syndrome*, ed. B. M. Hyde (Ottawa, ON: Nightingale Research Foundation, 1992), pp. 260–266.

5. K. P. May, S. G. West, et al., "Sleep Apnea in Male Patients With Fibromyalgia," *American Journal of Medicine* 94 (May 1993): 505–508.

6. *Johns Hopkins Medical Letter*, October 1994, pp. 5–6.

7. C. Thompson, D. Stanson, and A. Smith. "Seasonal Affective Disorder and Season-Dependent Abnormalities of Melatonin Supression by Light," *Lancet* 336 (1990): 703–706.

8. N. Rosenthal, "Diagnosis and Treatment of Seasonal Affective Disorder," *Journal of the American Medical Association* 270 (8 December 1993): 2717–2720.

9. D. O'Rourke, et al., "Treatment of Seasonal Depression With d-Fenluramine," *Journal of Clinical Psychiatry* 50 (1989): 343–347.

10. S. Ruhrmann and S. Kasper, "Seasonal Depression," *Medizinische Monatsschrift TUR Pharmazeuten* 15 (1992): 293–299.

11. J. Liebermann and D. S. Bell, "Serum Angiotensin–Converting Enzyme as a Marker for the Chronic Fatigue–Immune Dysfunction Syndrome: A Comparison to Serum Angiotensin–Converting Enzyme in Sarcordosis," *American Journal of Medicine* 95 (1993): 407–412.

12. Chronic Fatigue and Immune Dysfunction Syndrome Association of America, "Ft. Lauderdale Chronic Fatigue and Immune Dysfunction Syndrome Conference," 7–9 October 1994, conference handout.

13. J. Goldstein, "Fibromyalgia Syndrome: A Pain Modulation Disorder Related to Altered Limbic Function?" *Baillieres Clinical Rheumatology* 8 (November 1994): 777–800.

14. A. Gaby, "Potassium-Magnesium Aspartate: A Special Supplement for Tired People," *Nutrition and Healing*, October 1995, pp. 3–4, 11.

CHAPTER 7

1. J. M. Strosberg, "Is Fibrositis a Stress Disorder?" *Rheumatology for the Practicing Physician*, January 1989, p. 12.

2. H. Smythe, "Fibrositis Continues to Present Clinical Challenges," *Rheumatology for the Practicing Physician*, January 1989, pp. 13–14.

3. E. N. Griep, J. N. Boersma, et al., "Altered Reactivity of the HPA Axis in the Primary Fibromyalgia Syndrome," *Journal of Rheumatology* 20 (1993): 469–474.

APPENDIX A

1. E. M. Sternberg, "Hypoimmune Fatigue Syndromes: Disease of the Stress Response," *Journal of*

Rheumatology 20, editorial (1993): 418–421.

2. G. Neeck and W. Riedel, "Thyroid Function in Patients With Fibromyalgia Syndrome," *Journal of Rheumatology* 19 (1992): 1120–1122.

3. M. A. Demitrack, J. K. Dale, S. E. Strauss, L. Lave, S. J. Listwak, and M. J. Kreuss, "Evidence for Impaired Activation of the Hypothalamic-Pituitary-Adrenal Axis in Patients With Chronic Fatigue Syndrome," *Journal of Clinical Endocrinology and Metabolism* 73 (1991): 1223–1234.

4. A.M.O. Bakheit, P. O. Behan, T. G. Dinan, et al., "Possible Upregulation of Hypothalamic 5-HT Receptors in Patients With Postviral Fatigue Syndrome," *Boston Medical Journal* 304 (April 1992): 1010–1012.

5. E. N. Griep, J. N. Boersma, et al., "Altered Reactivity of the HPA Axis in the Primary Fibromyalgia Syndrome," *Journal of Rheumatology* 20 (1993): 469–474.

6. G. A. McCain and K. S. Tilbe, "Diurnal Hormone Variation in Fibromyalgia Syndrome and a Comparison With Rheumatoid Arthritis," *Journal of Rheumatology* 25 (1993): 469–474.

7. W. G. Crook, *The Yeast Connection* (Jackson, TN: Professional Books, 1983).

8. L. Galland, et al., "Giardia as a Cause of Chronic Fatigue," *Journal of Nutritional Medicine* 1 (1990): 27–31.

9. J. G. Travell and D. G. Simons, *Myofascial Pain and Dysfunction:*

The Trigger Point Manual, vol. 1 (Baltimore, MD: Williams & Wilkins, 1983), pp. 103–164.

10. R. K. Chandra, "Effect of Macro and Micro Nutrient Deficiencies and Excess on Immune Response," *Food Technology,* February 1985, pp. 91–93.

11. R. K. Chandra, et al., "NIH Workshop on Trace Element Regulation of Immunity and Infection," *Nutrition Research* 2 (1982): 721–733.

12. S. Chandra, et al., "Undernutrition Impairs Immunity," *Internal Medicine* 5 (December 1984): 85–99.

13. M. C. Talbott, "Pyridoxine Supplementation: Effect on Lymphocyte Responses in Elderly Persons," *American Journal of Clinical Nutrition* 46 (1987): 659–664.

14. S. N. Meydani, et al., "Vitamin E Supplementation Enhances Cell-Mediated Immunity in Healthy Elderly Subjects," *American Journal of Clinical Nutrition* 52 (1990): 557–563.

15. A. C. Chester, "Chronic Fatigue of Nasal Origin: Possible Confusion With Chronic Fatigue Syndrome," in *The Clinical and Scientific Basis of Myalgic Encephalitis and Chronic Fatigue Syndrome,* ed. B. M. Hyde (Ottawa, ON: Nightingale Research Foundation, 1992), pp. 260–266.

16. G. Faglia, et al., "Thyrotropin Secretion in Patients With Central Hypothyroidism," *Journal of Clinical Endocrinology and Metabolism* 48 (1979): 989–998.

17. N. R. Campbell, et al., "Ferrous Sulfate Reduces Thyroxine Efficacy in Patients With Hypothyroidism," *Annals of Internal Medicine* 117 (1992): 1010–1013.

18. M.J.A.J.M. Hoes, "Plasma Concentrations of Magnesium and Vitamin B1 in Alcoholism and Delirium Tremans," *Acta Psychiatrica Belgica* 81 (1981): 72–84.

19. T. Dyckner and P. O. Wester, "Ventricular Extrasystoles and Intracellular Electrolytes Before and After Potassium-Magnesium Infusions in Patients on Diuretic Treatment," *American Heart Journal* 97 (January 1979): 12–18.

20. G. E. Abraham and J. Fletchas, "Management of Fibromyalgia: Rationale for the Use of Magnesium and Malic Acid," *Journal of Nutritional Medicine* 3 (1992): 49–59.

21. D. C. Rushton, et al., "Letters to the Editor," *Lancet*, 22 June 1991, p. 1554.

22. T. F. Kirn, "Do Low Levels of Iron Affect Body's Ability to Regulate Temperature, Experience Cold?" *Journal of the American Medical Association*, 5 August 1988, p. 607.

23. J. Lindenbaum, E. B. Healton, et al., "Neuropsychiatric Disorders Caused by Cobalamin Deficiency in the Absence of Anemia or Macrocytoses," *New England Journal of Medicine* 318 (1988): 1720–1728.

24. J. Lindenbaum, et al., "Prevalence of Cobalamin Deficiency in the Framingham Elderly Population," *American Journal of Clinical Nutrition* 60 (1994): 2–11.

25. E. J. Norman, "Screening Elderly Populations for Cobalamin (Vitamin B12) Deficiency Using the Urinary Methylmalonic Acid Assay by Gas Chromotography Mass Spectometry," *American Journal of Medicine* 94 (June 1993): 589–594.

26. R. J. Deckelbaum, "ELISA More Accurate Than Microscopy for Giardia," *Infectious Diseases in Children*, October 1993, p. 30.

27. W. Jeffries, letter to author, 31 July 1993.

28. W. Jeffries, *Safe Uses of Cortisone*, monograph (Springfield, IL: Charles C. Thomas, 1981).

29. W. Jeffries, "Low Dose Glucocorticoid Therapy," *Archives of Internal Medicine* 119 (1967): 265–278.

30. E. Barrett-Connor, K. T. Khaw, and S.S.C. Yen, "A Prospective Study of DHEA, Mortality, and Cardiovascular Disease," *New England Journal of Medicine* 315 (1986): 1519–1524.

31. A. J. Morales, et al., "Effects of DHEA in Advancing Age," *Journal of Clinical Endocrinology and Metabolism* 78 (1994): 1360–1367.

32. I. A. Posner, "Treatment of Fibromyalgia Syndrome With IV Lidocaine: A Prospective, Randomized Pilot Study," *Journal of Musculoskeletal Pain* 2 (1994): 55–65.

33. J. Goldstein, *Betrayal by the Brain: The Neurologic Basis of Chronic Fatigue Syndrome, Fibromyalgia Syndrome and Related Neural Network Disorders* (Bing- hampton, NY: Haworth Press, 1996).

34. M. Brock, *Acta Neurochirurgica* 47, supplement (1990): 127– 128.

Bibliography

BOOKS

Braunwald, E., ed. *Harrisons Principles of Internal Medicine*, 11th ed. New York: McGraw-Hill, 1987.

Crook, W. G. *The Yeast Connection*. Jackson, TN: Professional Books, 1983.

Crook, W. G. *The Yeast Connection and the Woman*. Jackson, TN: Professional Books, 1995.

Dawson, D., and S. Sabin, ed. *Chronic Fatigue Syndrome*. Boston: Little, Brown and Company, 1993.

Gittleman, A. L. *Guess What Came to Dinner: Parasites and Your Health*. Garden City Park, NY: Avery Publishing Group, 1993.

Goldstein, J. *Betrayal by the Brain: The Neurologic Basis of Chronic Fatigue Syndrome, Fibromyalgia Syndrome and Related Neural Network Disorders*. Binghampton, NY: Haworth Press, 1996.

Hyde, B. M., ed. *The Clinical and Scientific Basis of Myalgic Encephalitis and Chronic Fatigue Syndrome*. Ottawa, ON: Nightingale Research Foundation, 1992.

Rogers, S. *Tired or Toxic*. Syracuse, NY: Prestige Publishing, 1990.

Travell, J. G., and D. G. Simons. *Myofascial Pain and Dysfunction: The Trigger Point Manual*, vol. 1. Baltimore, MD: Williams & Wilkins, 1983.

Trowell, H. C., ed. *Western Diseases: Their Emergence and Prevention.* Cambridge, MA: Harvard University Press, 1981.

ARTICLES

Abraham, G. E., and J. Fletchas. "Management of Fibromyalgia: Rationale for the Use of Magnesium and Malic Acid." *Journal of Nutritional Medicine* 3 (1992): 49–59.

Adams, F., J. R. Avesada, et al. "Neuropsychiatric Manifestations of Human Leukocyte Interferon Therapy in Patients With Cancer." *Journal of the American Medical Association* 252 (1984): 938–941.

Alexander, W. *Internal Medicine World Report,* 1–14 January 1995, p. 32.

Anderson, R. A., et al. "Chromium and Hypoglycemia." *American Journal of Clinical Nutrition* 41, abstract (April 1985): 841.

Aoki, T., H. Miyakoshi, et al. "Low NK Syndrome and Its Relationship to Chronic Fatigue Syndrome." *Clinical Immunology and Immunopathology* 69 (December 1993): 253–265.

Archard, L. E., N. E. Bowles, P. O. Behan, et al. "Postviral Fatigue Syndrome Persistence of Enterovirus RNA in Muscle and Elevated Creatine Kinase." *Journal of the Royal Society of Medicine* 81 (1988): 326–329.

Avorn, J. "Reduction of Bacteriuria and Pyuria After Ingestion of Cranberry Juice." *Journal of the American Medical Association* 271 (1994): 751–754.

Bakheit, A.M.O., P. O. Behan, et al. "Abnormal Arginine-Vasopressin Secretion and Water Metabolism in Patients With Post-Viral Fatigue Syndrome." *Acta Neurologica Scandinavica* 87 (1993): 234–238.

Bakheit, A.M.O., P. O. Behan, T. G. Dinan, et al. "Possible Upregulation of Hypothalamic 5-HT Receptors in Patients With Postviral Fatigue Syndrome." *Boston Medical Journal* 304 (April 1992): 1010–1012.

Barker, E., S. F. Fujimura, et al. "Immunologic Abnormalities Associated With Chronic Fatigue Syndrome." *Clinical Infectious Diseases* 18, supplement 1 (1994): 5136–5141.

Barrett-Connor, E., R. T. Khaw, and S. C. Yen. "A Prospective Study of DHEA, Mortality and Cardiovascular Disease." *New England Journal of Medicine* 315 (1986): 1519–1524.

Beck, W. S. "Cobalamin and the Nervous System." *New England Journal of Medicine* 318, editorial (1988): 1752–1754.

Bennet, R. B., S. R. Clark, et al. "Low Levels of Somatomedin C in Patients With the Fibromyalgia Syndrome." *Arthritis and Rheumatism* 35 (1992): 1113–1116.

Bennett, R. M., R. A. Gatter, et al. "Cyclobenzaprine Versus Placebo in Fibromyalgia." *Arthritis and Rheumatism* 31 (December 1988): 1535–1542.

Boyne, R. *Journal of Nutrition* 116 (1982): 816–822.

Brock, M. *Acta Neurochirurgica* 47, supplement (1990): 127–128.

Campbell, N. R., et al. "Ferrous Sulfate Reduces Thyroxine Efficacy in Patients With Hypothyroidism." *Annals of Internal Medicine* 117 (1992): 1010–1013.

Chandra, R. K. "Effect of Macro and Micro Nutrient Deficiencies and Excess on Immune Response." *Food Technology*, February 1985, pp. 91–93.

Chandra, R. K., et al. "NIH Workshop on Trace Element Regulation of Immunity and Infection." *Nutrition Research* 2 (1982): 721–733.

Chandra, S., et al. "Undernutrition Impairs Immunity." *Internal Medicine* 5 (December 1984): 85–99.

Cuneo, R. C., F. Salomen, et al. "GH Treatment in Growth Hormone Deficient Adults," part II: "Effects on Exercise Performance." *Journal of Applied Physiology* 70 (1991): 695–700.

Darnell, L. S. "Abstract 21." *American Journal of Clinical Nutrition*, supplement.

Deckelbaum, R. J. "ELISA More Accurate Than Microscopy for Giardia." *Infectious Diseases in Children*, October 1993, p. 30.

Demitrack, M. A., J. K. Dale, S. E. Strauss, L. Lave, S. J. Listwak, and M. J. Kreuss. "Evidence for Impaired Activation of the

Hypothalamic-Pituitary-Adrenal Axis in Patients With Chronic Fatigue Syndrome." *Journal of Clinical Endocrinology and Metabolism* 73 (1991): 1223–1234.

Dressing, H., and D. Riemann. "Insomnia: Are Valerian/Melissa Combinations of Equal Value to Benzodiazepine?" *Therapiewoche* 42 (1992): 726–736.

Dyckner, T., and P. O. Wester. "Ventricular Extrasystoles and Intracellular Electrolytes Before and After Potassium-Magnesium Infusions in Patients on Diuretic Treatment." *American Heart Journal* 97 (January 1979): 12–18.

Eaton, S. B. "Paleolithic Nutrition." *New England Journal of Medicine* 312 (31 January 1985): 283–289.

Edman, J., et al. "Zinc Status in Women With Recurrent Vulvovaginal Candidiasis." *American Journal of Obstetrics and Gynecology* 155 (1986): 1082–1088.

Faglia, G., et al. "Thyrotropin Secretion in Patients With Central Hypothyroidism." *Journal of Clinical Endocrinology and Metabolism* 48 (1979): 989–998.

Gaby, A. "Potassium-Magnesium Aspartate: A Special Supplement for Tired People." *Nutrition and Healing*, October 1995, pp. 3–4, 11.

Galland, L., et al. "Giardia as a Cause of Chronic Fatigue." *Journal of Nutritional Medicine* 1 (1990): 27–31.

Gambrell, R. D. *Consultant*, July 1994, pp. 1047–1057.

Gatter, R. A. "Pharmacotherapeutics in Fibromyalgia." *American Journal of Medicine* 81, supplement 3A (29 September 1986): 63–66.

Goldenberg, D. L. "Fibromyalgia Syndrome." *Journal of the American Medical Association* 257 (1987): 2782–2787.

Goldstein, J. "Fibromyalgia Syndrome: A Pain Modulation Disorder Related to Altered Limbic Function?" *Baillieres Clinical Rheumatology* 8 (November 1994): 777–800.

Griep, E. N., J. N. Boersma, et al. "Altered Reactivity of the HPA Axis in the Primary Fibromyalgia Syndrome." *Journal of Rheumatology* 20 (1993): 469–474.

Halpin, D., and S. Wessely. "VP-1 Antigen in Chronic Postviral Fatigue Syndrome." *Lancet*, 1989, pp. 1028–1029.

Hoes, M.J.A.J.M. "Plasma Concentrations of Magnesium and Vitamin B₁ in Alcoholism and Delirium Tremans." *Acta Psychiatrica Belgica* 81 (1981): 72–84.

Holmes, G. P., J. E. Kaplan, et al. "Chronic Fatigue Syndrome: A Working Case Definition." *Annals of Internal Medicine* 108 (1988): 387–389.

Jeffries, W. "Low Dose Glucocorticoid Therapy." *Archives of Internal Medicine* 119 (1967): 265–278.

Jenkins, J. S. "The Role of Oxytocin: Present Concepts." *Clinical Endocrinology* 34 (1991): 515–525.

Johns Hopkins Medical Letter, October 1994, pp. 5–6.

Jorgensen, J.O.L., S. A. Pedersen, et al. "Long Term GH Treatment in Growth Hormone Deficient Adults." *Acta Endocrinol (Copenhagen)* 125 (1991): 449–453.

Karnaze, D. S., et al. "Low Serum Cobalmin Levels in Primary Degenerative Dementia: Do Some Patients Harbor Atypical Cobalmin Deficiency States?" *Archives of Internal Medicine* 147 (1987): 429–431.

Kennes, B., et al. "Effect of Vitamin C Supplements on Cell-Mediated Immunity in Old People." *Gerontology* 29 (1983): 305–310.

Kirn, T. F. "Do Low Levels of Iron Affect Body's Ability to Regulate Temperature, Experience Cold?" *Journal of the American Medical Association* 260 (5 August 1988): 607.

Lakshmanad, F. L., et al. "Magnesium Intakes and Balances." *American Journal of Clinical Nutrition* 40, supplement (December 1984): 1380–1389.

Liebermann, J., and D. S. Bell. "Serum Angiotensin–Converting Enzyme as a Marker for the Chronic Fatigue–Immune Dysfunction Syndrome: A Comparison to Serum Angiotensin–Converting Enzyme in Sarcordosis." *American Journal of Medicine* 95 (1993): 407–412.

Lindenbaum, J., et al. "Prevalence of Cobalamin Deficiency in the Framingham Elderly Population." *American Journal of Clinical Nutrition* 60 (1994): 2–11.

Lindenbaum, J., E. B. Healton, et al. "Neuropsychiatric Disorders Caused by Cobalamin Deficiency in the Absence of Anemia or Macrocytoses." *New England Journal of Medicine* 318 (1988): 1720–1728.

Marchesani, R. B. "Critical Antiviral Pathway Deficient in Chronic Fatigue Syndrome Patients." *Infectious Disease News,* August 1993, p. 4.

Marston, R. M., and B. B. Peterkin. "Nutrient Content of the National Food Supply." *National Food Review,* Winter 1980, pp. 21–25.

May, K. P., S. G. West, et al. "Sleep Apnea in Male Patients With Fibromyalgia." *American Journal of Medicine* 94 (May 1993): 505–508.

McCain, G. A., and K. S. Tilbe. "Diurnal Hormone Variation in Fibromyalgia Syndrome and a Comparison With Rheumatoid Arthritis." *Journal of Rheumatology* 25 (1993): 469–474.

McGauley, G. A. "Quality of Life Assessment Before and After Growth Hormone Treatment in Adults With GH Deficiency." *Acta Paediatrica Scandinavica* 356, supplement (1989): 70–72.

Meikle, A. W., et al. "Adrenal Androgen Secretion and Biologic Effects." *Endocrine and Metabolic Clinics of North America* 20, June 1991, pp. 381–421.

Mertz, W., ed. "Beltsville 1 Year Dietary Intake Survey." *American Journal of Clinical Nutrition* 40, supplement (December 1984): 1323–1403.

Meydani, S. N., et al. "Vitamin E Supplementation Enhances Cell-Mediated Immunity in Healthy Elderly Subjects." *American Journal of Clinical Nutrition* 52 (1990): 557–563.

Morales, A. J., et al. "Effects of DHEA in Advancing Age." *Journal of Clinical Endocrinology and Metabolism* 78 (1994): 1360–1367.

Neeck, G., and W. Riedel. "Thyroid Function in Patients With

Fibromyalgia Syndrome." *Journal of Rheumatology* 19 (1992): 1120–1122.

Nelson, J. H. "Wheat—Its Processing and Utilization." *American Journal of Clinical Nutrition* 41, supplement (May 1985): 1070–1076.

Norman, E. J. "Screening Elderly Populations for Cobalamin (Vitamin B_{12}) Deficiency Using the Urinary Methylmalonic Acid Assay by Gas Chromotography Mass Spectometry." *American Journal of Medicine* 94 (June 1993): 589–594.

O'Rourke, D., et al. "Treatment of Seasonal Depression With d-Fenluramine." *Journal of Clinical Psychiatry* 50 (1989): 343–347.

Parker, L. N. "Control of Adrenal Androgen Secretion." *Endocrine and Metabolic Clinics of North America* 20 (June 1991): 401–421.

Posner, I. A. "Treatment of Fibromyalgia Syndrome With IV Lidocaine: A Prospective, Randomized Pilot Study." *Journal of Musculoskeletal Pain* 2 (1994): 55–65.

Price, R. K., C. S. North, et al. "Estimating the Presence of Chronic Fatigue Syndrome in the Community." *Public Health Reports* 107 (September–October 1992): 514–522.

Quesada, J. R., M. Talpaz, et al. "Clinical Toxicity of Interferon in Cancer Patients: A Review." *Journal of Clinical Oncology* 4 (February 1986): 234–243.

Reid, G. "Implantation of Lactobacillus Casei Var Rhamnosus Into Vagina." *Lancet* 344, letter (29 October 1994): 1229.

Rogers, S. "Chemical Sensitivity: Breaking the Paralyzing Paradigm," part I. *Internal Medicine World Report*, vol. 7, no. 3, p. 1.

Rogers, S. "Chemical Sensitivity: Breaking the Paralyzing Paradigm," part II. *Internal Medicine World Report*, vol. 7, no. 6, pp. 8, 21–31.

Rosenthal, N. "Diagnosis and Treatment of Seasonal Affective Disorder." *Journal of the American Medical Association* 270 (8 December 1993): 2717–2720.

Rowe, P. C., I. Bole-Hoiaighah, J. S. Kan, and H. Calkins. "Is

Neurally Mediated Hypotension an Unrecognized Cause of Chronic Fatigue?" *Lancet* 345 (11 March 1995): 623–624.

Ruhrmann, S., and S. Kasper. "Seasonal Depression." *Medizinische Monatsschrift TUR Pharmazeuten* 15 (1992): 293–299.

Rushton, D. C., et al. "Letters to the Editor." *Lancet*, 22 June 1991, p. 1554.

Schroeder, H. A. "Loss of Vitamins and Trace Minerals Resulting From Processing and Preservation of Foods." *American Journal of Clinical Nutrition* 24 (May 1971): 562–573.

Seelig, M. S. "The Requirement of Magnesium by the Normal Adult." *American Journal of Clinical Nutrition* 14 (June 1964): 342–390.

Simons, D. G. "Myofascial Pain Syndrome Due to Trigger Points." *International Rehabilitation Medicine Association Monograph Series* 1 (November 1987).

Smythe, H. "Fibrositis Continues to Present Clinical Challenges." *Rheumatology for the Practicing Physician*, January 1989, pp. 13–14.

Sternberg, E. M. "Hypoimmune Fatigue Syndromes: Disease of the Stress Response." *Journal of Rheumatology* 20, editorial (1993): 418–421.

Strauss, S. E., S. Fritz, J. K. Dale, B. Gould, and W. Strober. "Lymphocyte Phenotype and Function in Chronic Fatigue Syndrome." *Journal of Clinical Immunology* 13 (January 1993): 30–40.

Strosberg, J. M. "Is Fibrositis a Stress Disorder?" *Rheumatology for the Practicing Physician*, January 1989, p. 12.

Talbott, M. C. "Pyridoxine Supplementation: Effect on Lymphocyte Responses in Elderly Persons." *American Journal of Clinical Nutrition* 46 (1987): 659–664.

Teitelbaum, J., and B. Bird. "Effective Treatment of Severe Chronic Fatigue: A Report of a Series of 64 Patients." *Journal of Musculoskeletal Pain* 3 (1995): 91–110.

Thompson, C., D. Stanson, and A. Smith. "Seasonal Affective

Disorder and Season-Dependent Abnormalities of Melatonin Supression by Light." *Lancet* 336 (1990): 703–706.

Travell, J. *Archives of Physical Medicine and Rehabilitation* 62 (1981): 100–106.

Vance, M. L. "Hypopituitarism." *New England Journal of Medicine* 330: 1651–1662.

Wakefield, D., A. Lloyd, and J. Dwyer. "Human Herpes Virus 6 and Myalgic Encephalomyelitis." *Lancet*, 1988, p. 1059.

Walter, T., et al. *American Journal of Clinical Nutrition* 44 (1986): 877–882.

Yousef, G. E., E. J. Bell, et al. "Chronic Enterovirus Infection in Patients With Postviral Fatigue Syndrome." *Lancet*, 1988, pp. 146–147.

Zelissen, P.M.J., et al. "Effect of Glucocorticord Replacement Therapy on Bone Mineral Density in Patients With Addison's Disease." *Annals of Internal Medicine* 120 (1994): 207–210.

MISCELLANEOUS MATERIALS

Chronic Fatigue and Immune Dysfunction Syndrome Association of America. "Ft. Lauderdale Chronic Fatigue and Immune Dysfunction Syndrome Conference," 7–9 October 1994. Conference handout.

Jeffries, W. *Safe Uses of Cortisone*. Monograph. Springfield, IL: Charles C. Thomas, 1981.

Procter and Gamble Pharmaceuticals, inhouse research data.

Simons, D. G. "Myofascial Pain Syndrome Due to Trigger Points." *International Rehabilitation Medicine Association Monograph Series* 1 (November 1987).

Permission Credits

The cartoons on pages 4 and 14 (top and bottom) are reprinted with the permission of Scott Arthur Maseur.

The "Updated CDC Criteria for Chronic Fatigue Syndrome" on page 7 is adapted from the *Annals of Internal Medicine* 121 (14 December 1994). Used with permission.

The cartoon on page 24 is from *Punch*, © 1989.

The cartoons on pages 40 (top), 76, and 81 are reprinted with the permission of Edgar Argo.

The cartoon on page 40 (bottom) is reprinted with the special permission of the North America Syndicate.

The cartoon on page 52 is reprinted with the special permission of King Features Syndicate.

The "Criteria for Fibromyalgia" and illustration on page 54 and the "American College of Rheumatology 1990 Criteria for the Classification of Fibromyalgia" on pages 93–94 are adapted from F. Wolfe, et al., "The American College of Rheumatology 1990 Criteria for the Classification of Fibromyalgia: Report of the Multicenter Criteria Committee," *Arthritis and Rheumatology* 33 (1990). Used with permission.

The cartoon on page 60 is reprinted with the permission of Tribune Media Services.

The cartoon on page 82 is by Swan, © 1989.

"Effective Treatment of Severe Chronic Fatigue: A Report of a Serie

Index